Surya Namascaredy-Pants

A Prana Weinberg Mystery

By
Margaret France

Published by kraft-o-matix
kraft-o-matix
Slavin and West Slavin
Peshastin, Washington

ISBN 978-0692578766 (kraft-o-matix)

Sunday

"It's Weinberg, e-i, comma, PI comma, MA comma, PHR."

"Shanti R! Jasmine tea and chia pudding!" A thirtyish blur of bright leggings rushes past our table, clearly under chia-ed.

"Did you get that, Josh? PI, then MA, then PHR."

"Don't you think you should put the 'PI' part last?"

"What? Why?"

"I don't know, just seems more . . . Magnum." I don't know if I should be happy or sad that a hero from my childhood has been gone long enough to be revived as a camp idol for Josh, who has the kind of facial scraggle that begs to be carded for cigarettes.

"Okay, let's see it both ways." I'm not wearing a Hawaiian shirt or growing a mustache. In fact, despite our differences in plumbing and age, I really fancy myself more of a Rockford. Weinberg Files? Of course they both had terrible cars for cover—a red Ferrari on an island? If I wasn't commodore of a fleet of unsalable Honda Accords I don't know if I would have become a licensed private investigator. But I am, I did, and now people need to know who I am on the internet.

"You know you have a Google problem, right?"

The half muffin emerges from its small waxy cover. The owner carelessly shoved it in and directly out of his Chrome messenger bag. Now it falls in slow motion. Fancy's ears perk up at full speed, almost as quickly as I squeeze out from behind the counter and sprint to the other side of the door. "No Fancy, not for you!" I glance at the patio dwellers. "She's gluten-free." They shrug. I know, I should be sitting outside with her. I give her a treat, "Good job, Fance. Just a couple more minutes, kay?"

"When you put 'weinberg' and 'investigation' in, you get—this." Josh's screen fills with news items. My last name might as well be "Ponzi," for all the trial reports, thumbnails from perp walks, and excoriating commentary that sits in miniature, just a click away. I am a few keystrokes from disaster, literally. "Yeah, so I know you said you didn't want a picture on the site, which I get, but maybe, like your first name?" I chew on this suggestion. It tastes like my lower lip, dryer and saltier than I imagined. "Like this: 'Prana Weinberg, MA, PHR, PI Investigations.' It's your name, right? And it automatically says, toe-tally different kind of Weinberg! Not remotely Barry Weinberg!" I am stilled by the exhaustion of being on the verge of explaining something for the millionth time that should be completely obvious. I am in control.

"Ehm, can I see it mocked both ways? We don't need to go live until the beginning of next week."

"If you want to spend the money."

"It's just another homepage, right? The rest wouldn't make any difference."

"Well, every link goes right back to the homepage, which you could just call 'home' and then it doesn't matter, but it's sort of nice to have a banner all the way through the site that leads back, so yeah, I guess it does matter on the other pages, too. Maybe take another couple hours?" Another couple hours of Josh's time will run me at least two hundred dollars. It's incredible how much I have to pay myself so that I can afford to pay other people to pay themselves so they can afford to pay eight-hundred dollars for their third of the seven hundred square feet that constitutes the realization of all their Midwestern liberal arts college dreams. Move to the Bay Area. Be with your people. Be with them after they move to Bay Point, which seems like it should be close but is really, really far from everything. Be with them after they move to the South Bay, where the most notable cultural feature involves a gas station with a cook in the back who will batter and fry anything purchased it on-site, including a tire pressure gauge, because you asked because what else in the South Bay. Be with them after they start spending their weekends raising money to build something called a "Kilt-A-Whirl" on a place called the Playa, so that men can wear skirts that fly up as it spins, making for a truly terrible series of Instagrams so that even though the "Kilt-A-Whirl" will be destroyed after less than five windslapped, dirt-etched days and nights, the blurry members will ride forever. Josh looks tired.

"Do it."

———

"So the look on his face?" Tammy's eyes illuminate with a sparkle just this side of manic. She gallantly lets me take the shady side of the patio table for our meeting without saying a word, either forgetting to kid me about my sun paranoia—certainly her right, but she seems to think her brown skin is a lead apron in the face UVs A and B—or so excited to get the low-down on the delivery of her divorce papers in person that she just can't be bothered to pick on me. I thought I needed an office to put out a shingle as a PI, but it's surprising how happy clients are to just meet up at a coffee shop. The fact that all my clients so far are people I already know might be a factor there, too.

———

"Well, yeah, he was pretty surprised."

"But, pissed, right? Really pissed? Minor-to-moderately self-shittingly pissed?"

I am not familiar enough with men's anatomy to know if that is genuinely plausible. It's one of those follow-up questions I wanted to ask when Doug Guintoli explained to me how that scene in *Silence of Lambs* works, where he's dancing in the mirror and he doesn't have any junk. I was forthright enough in the eleventh grade to inquire, but too shy to, well, *probe* Doug, and now, while I'm not entirely sure what happens when a man pees and takes a dump at the same time, I'm fairly certain that's not what Tammy's soon-to-be ex-husband did when I served him. Still, it is my professional duty to make her feel good about hiring me.

"I think he farted, like, a startled fart. I mean, I know you wanted me to really process his reaction, but Fancy was not staying. She has a much better sense of smell than we do, you know." Fancy, alerted by the sound of her name but already mildly distressed by the time elapsed between the invocation of her Fancy-ness and production of treats, cocks her head impatiently acknowledging her superior olfactory sensitivity. "Who's a good dog who serves papers and makes men fart in terror? That's yooooouuuuu, Fancy!" I pull a treat from my bag, which Fancy accepts with all the fanfare and gratitude of a bus patron taking a transfer.

The patio at ROOZ is more imaginary than actual, a couple of black metal tables and some rickety wooden chairs that wouldn't have passed muster with the students, freelancers and book groups inside without a napkin wadded up under a leg. Outside, expectations go down, and for Fancy it was a lovely spot, with a bowl of water generally full, never stale, never lukewarm from the sun.

"Okay, I'm sorry. Just go through it one more time."

"I've got my backpack, right? And he's coming out of the BART and I bump him. He apologizes, and I realize it's open—"

"Right, all the sudden. Love it!"

"—and I hand him Fancy's leash."

"Yeah." Tammy's eyes are shut now. She sucked down her pint glass of coffee so quickly that the image she relishes behind her eyes right now must be shaky.

"I reach in and grab the papers and say, 'trade ya.'"

"Trade ya!"

"And then I say, Michael Cho, you've been served."

"Yes! Again! God, I wish you offered like, a service, where if I pay more, you film it."

"Do you know, off-hand, if that would be, like, legal?"

"Prana, you know better than to ask me shit like that. I'm in the inspector general's office. I can tell you all about audits and compliance, but like actual regular-people law stuff? It's long gone."

"I'm kidding. I don't give a shit if it's legal, but I suspect it might make me a bad person, person, you know, enabling people to perseverate over this stuff."

Tammy gives me a sour smile. "'Perseverate?' Look at you with your fancy words." Fancy looks up at Tammy, a genie from a bottle who has come to take wishes, not give them. "Is this your way of telling me you like my scone, sweetie?"

"No!" I put my hand over Tammy's before she can offer a morsel to Fancy's impatient maw. "Fancy, if you stop begging I'll give you a treat! A gluten-free treat like you're supposed have, okay?"

"Aww," Tammy smiles. "A second there, I thought maybe you were putting the moves on me now that I'm so much closer to being single."

"Sorry."

"You're not really my type, but anything for a discount. Three hundred dollars may not be a lot of money to you, but I work for the city."

"It took three tries. I know it seems like a lot, but that's with the friend discount. The way the hourly breaks down . . ."

"No, I trust you, it's just, with the divorce . . ."

"You know what, don't pay me now. I know where to find you. Maybe we can work something out."

"Is this flirting? I know Iris left, but I'm the one with the real divorce, don't play."

"You were married way too long if you think this is flirting. But if it makes you feel better, I'm sure you'll be able to do me a favor some day, Tammy, or should I say, Lieutenant Cho."

"I'm getting rid of that, but not the lieutenant part, so yeah, hit me up."

Monday

"C'mon Fancy, in or out." I will not be one of those people who has lived alone for so long that they habitually leave the bathroom door open so make up your mind, door's a shuttin'. Decorum for one seems like something worth maintaining. Despite giving up on eating anything but popcorn and Brussels sprouts for dinner, I still want to live a life that can withstand the view from a second (well, third, HELLO FANCY!) pair of eyes. Hall and Oates? Work ring. At least I'm already in an ergonomic seated position.

"Weinberg Investigations."

"Can I speak to Prana?"

"One moment." I drop my voice back to its natural habitat, a hair north of gullet. "Prana Weinberg."

"Hi, um, I've never done this before. Like, investigated? But, so, my studio? I think someone's maybe, borrowing money? And I just need to know who, so we can work out, like, a plan?"

"I'm sorry, with whom am I speaking?"

"Ha, sorry, my name is Aria Butler. I own Yoginitini, on Telegraph?"

"Right."

"We're the only studio in town with a liquor license? For now . . ." I can almost hear fingers crossing on the other end of the line.

"Have you called the police?"

"It's complicated. So the last time I called was when my bike was stolen? And I had to fill out a form online? Then Tai saw it on Craig's list, and I tried to talk to someone again, like, this is *my* bike, these are real criminals, how am I supposed to deal with them, right?"

"So . . ."

"Fuck them." And Aria Butler finally makes a declarative statement.

"Look, I think we'd both be more comfortable discussing this in person. I can certainly set up surveillance of your studio, but it might work best if you familiarize me with the situation on site, probably after hours. Since you might not want to meet a stranger alone in those circumstances, we can meet for coffee or tea beforehand and I can let you know what kind of operation I run."

"Oh no, I don't need to meet you first, Prana."

"Are you a referral?"

"No but, I mean I just feel, like, comfortable already?" If there were an infographic word map of my entire lifetime of utterances, looming even larger than "Fancy" or "Iris" or even "mine" would be the five words I'm thinking so loudly I'm surprised they haven't already fallen out and into the ether: I did *not* name myself.

Aria, oblivious to my silent annoyance with my parents and the way they spent the seventies, continues, unfettered, as if I were still listening. Which I should be. This is not sound investigation, or use of my human resources. It is private, though, here in the bathroom.

"Like, come on the police are going to care? I mean, you can only get them to come out if the robbery is like, happening right then?"

"Right." The beleaguered Oakland PD has wrung out three chiefs in two years. No property crime not in progress was worth sending a unit. In fact, it takes more and more just to get arrested in Oakland, something that, when I moved here after college, would have seemed like a dream come true. A dozen years later the cops really have stopped caring. I benefit, not because I can stroll down Broadway smoking a joint, but because the fissure between the services citizens expect from their police force and the limited assistance the OPD can actually provide leaves a little room for the private sector to take over.

So much room for me in there, but nothing to get smug about. This gorgeous city, the bright side of the Bay, where the marine layer is just a tourist, is also where the legalization of pot left legions of former dealers to make money with guns instead of ganja, where telephone poles are covered in homemade signs begging for the return of a MacBook, dates of the neighborhood watch meeting, and exhortations not to "walk and talk"—you might as well hold a couple fifties up to your ear while yelling, "I can't feel my hands!"

Aria Butler continues. "But it's not even like a robbery. I've just dropped in and I see the pouch, like bulging, and then I'm back at night and it's kinda light and the numbers work out with the sign-ins, but." I hear a deep cleansing breath. "And then sometimes. Sometimes there's too much money. Too much!" I hear a slow release of air, barely this side of a sigh. "I just need to know, if there's anyone, I can't—I mean, anyone, anyone I should maybe reach out to? My husband, he's mostly at our place in Los Gatos, and he says that the guys his company uses just wouldn't care about this. But you. *Prana.* I just have this feeling. I think, Prana, you are exactly what we need."

Whatever Iris thought about the environment, desirable urban housing, and the efficacy of Craig's List as a means of liquefying assets, I maintain that the only sensible thing to do with three late-model Honda Accords in gold, silver, and cream is to name them after the Gabor sisters and to never, ever pay to park them. I give Zsa Zsa a quick once-over before setting off down Telegraph to get my introduction to the East Bay's only bar and yoga studio. No valuables or change visible, not even an empty water bottle. I used to leave her unlocked to save the windows. Then some kids threw an old TV at her until her rear windshield shattered. My neighbor said it took them three tries. Zsa Zsa's no quitter. I own three Honda Accords, and none have been stolen; statistically I can't complain, as exasperating as it is to keep the Gabor sisters ahead of the street-cleaners.

In the semi-Korean, semi-Hipster district, across from the red Mama Buzz sign, I see the sign for Yoginitini: spare, no caps, parentheses encasing the "tini" part, as if it were an afterthought, or optional, which I suppose it is. Aria Butler cracks the outside door before I can ring in.

"Prana!" My current position, within her smooth, lightly tanned embrace, gives me a lousy prospect for taking in Aria Butler in all her Aria Butlerness. Especially since this embrace has already gone beyond its natural end to something else. She now seems to be trying to press up against my chest, seeking a chakra or maybe a banda, but succeeding only in smooshing her exuberant Bs against my exhausted As. Still, even from this compromised vantage, she is clearly the Aria of her YouTube videos, blonde hair spilling out from deep brown roots, eyes hinting at her Japanese heritage while the set of her nose and cheekbones suggest a greatest hits of Eastern European phenotypes, the rest of her body splitting the difference. The gold tint of her skin reminds me of the inside of a Milky Way, not that my allusion would mean anything to her. The toned shoulders giving way to tastefully defined biceps and delicate wrists suggest that she hasn't seen the inside of a Milky Way for decades.

"Aria. Blessed to meet you." She still grips my forearms, which would seem pretty hairy by comparison, if one of us weren't wearing, you know, people clothes. Aria, now that she has stepped back, is wearing yellow boy shorts and a plum-colored racerback bra, each with just enough contrasting swirl screened onto one side to graduate it from underwear to outerwear, though the line is so fine, the entire ensemble should be sent to summer school.

Shaking hands at this point would not only be redundant but insulting, like ordering Pizza Hut while lined up at Zachary's. She lets go of me only to direct me to the studio, taking me down a short hallway into a small, tasteful lobby with cubbies and bathrooms, and finally, after I slide out of my yellow boat-mocs, through rough-hewn double doors.

"Namaste. This is Yoginitini." The studio she ushers me into deserves the pride that creeps into her voice as she says its name. I dimly recall its previous life as a Korean karaoke parlor, but I would have a tough time selling anyone on that version of the past now. The space has been opened up as a loft-like area, with a raised bar on one end whose platform could double as a stage for demonstrating poses before a particularly crowded class. The room is large enough that it would take at least thirty students before the platform would be remotely necessary. Aside from the doors, the entire wall is mirrored, reflecting the light streaming in from the two-story windows. While the hallway and lobby seem a little small and claustrophobic, the studio is spacious. She must have taken out the entire floor above it to get them so high.

The mirrors, lightly frosted, give shapes more than details, as if designed for yoginis in the witness protection program. Refurbished wine barrels hold rolled mats in primary colors, bold bougie versions of the cups of crayons meant to keep kids from screaming at family restaurants. Next to them sit a broad shelf that looks like the same slats reconfigured, offering bricks, straps, towels and blankets, and then double doors—probably closet space. The bar was a burled, polished hardwood perched on a platform covered in a mosaic of mirrored glass, frosted, like the glass wall. The effect is somewhere between a health spa and a coke den, with a little sugary breakfast cereal thrown in, especially with Aria alone at the center of it all, possibly grrreat, also possibly a silly rabbit.

"This space, it's incredible. I was actually in here before, and . . ."

"Oh yeah, that was fun, but pretty grody. We took out all the walls, and then knocked out the apartment above the studio space."

"I was gonna say . . ."

"Yeah, only way to get the light, the feel, the air. Do you practice?"

"Yoga? Not really."

"Do you drink?"

It is two-fifteen on a Monday afternoon. I am a private eye. "Yep!"

"Super!" I follow Aria up to the bar. She chops, muddles, mixes, keeping up a cheerful patter throughout—where the wood from the bar came from, whose barrels she's using to store the mats, where she found her carpenter. Only when she presents us both with pink-tinged beverages, served up, do I remember that she never actually asked me what I wanted. I sip—grapefruit, rosemary, something maybe ginger in the background?

"This is good. Wow. Very herby."

"I can't tell you exactly what's in it, but it's our signature, the Bakhtini."

I take another sip. "Well it's certainly stimulating my dialogic imagination!"

"Sorry?"

"Oh—what, what does the name mean?" It suddenly occurs to me that designing a drinks menu to appeal to retired graduate students—a post-modern, a Marx julep, a Hegel Wallbanger, a Cixous on the beach—might not have been Aria's intent.

"Seriously, Prana? Your name is 'Prana' and you don't know what bakhti is? You are adorable." My cheeks feel warm. I am maybe a pinky into this Bakhtini and decide a breath is in order. She has not hired me yet.

"Yeah, that's funny. My parents, they were sort of into, oh, all kinds of stuff in the seventies."

"Seekers?"

"Umm. Yes. They named me Prana because that's what they really wanted. But I was, you know, a child, not a life force or anything like that. If I were born today, they would probably name me 'Compound Interest' or 'Tylenol 4.'"

"Oh, so you're not, like . . ."

"I didn't name myself, no."

Aria intuits that she is about to step in something and proceeds with all the caution I would expect from someone who makes her living in her bare feet.

Before she can follow up, or apologize, or offer me another drink, it occurs to me that I need a job. "I'm an open book, Aria. I want you to feel comfortable with me because I will need total access to your business to get to the bottom of this . . . employee theft? That was your concern on the phone."

"I hate that word, theft, I mean, what do we own? Do we own, like, money?" I struggle to set my face into some sort of neutral, commiserative arrangement. There is nothing unsnarky for me to say. Instead of responding, I attempt listening eyes. Aria continues, confirming either the triumph of my masquerade or her complete lack of interest in my opinion. "This studio, this, team, well, we're like . . ."

"A family?"

"Yes, and if anything's going on, people borrowing from the studio, I don't want it to be a secret, I don't want a minor setback for one of us to turn into something toxic for the whole studio, like a cold just turning into cancer." And neither of us were health science majors, but I won't correct her there, either, not just because I want this gig, but the sincerity with she talks about her employees demands respect. She doesn't care about the money, which, fair enough: if I were married to a Silicon Valley venture capitalist whose internet bubble forgot to burst, I might see the fiduciary inconsistencies in my small business as Aria does. She takes a deep breath. "Someone's telling me with money that they need something else, that their spirits are hungry. I just want to know who."

"Well . . . so I guess the register . . ." I take in the space again, noting the luxuriant hanging ferns, the broad wood slats on the floor, but nothing that looks like the heart of a retail establishment. "Did I walk by it in the lobby?"

"No, no. We use Square, and this." She holds up a silky embroidered pouch. "The register I tried, the display was just, super bright? So there was all this gross light? So I thought, put it in the lobby, but then someone has to work the front while the bar's open."

"You don't have a door man? In this neighborhood?" You can buzz clients into a studio, but buzzing buzzed bar patrons seems a little too speakeasy, even for Oakland.

"I do, but not by choice. My husband, he insists, so it's part of his team, or whoever he contracts, I don't really know how it works. They're all super-sweet guys, but they don't work for me, they work for him, so I can't very well make them responsible for ringing up the bar tabs and stuff. So we have an iPad and the pouch for the classes and the bar."

"Yes, you mentioned the pouch on the phone. And you also said that sometimes there might be too much money?"

"Ohmigosh, well, Prana, it's so important to me, I mean, if you take this job, that you come to some classes. Tai, Michelle, Faryn, they are so talented, just creative, gorgeous spirits. And they do everything. If I didn't own this studio I would still, just, camp here, because the people?"

"And you think they might be, um, stealing or giving you money?"

"Oh yeah, that's where I was going. I'm just in and out a lot, but I make time to take classes from everyone. Make time—I want to take their classes. It's not really about business at all really. So when I'm taking someone's class, you know, I sort of see what the set-up is, but I don't want to seem like I'm checking up on them or anything. I'm not at all. But I have noticed the pouch bulging and then I come in at the end of the day and there's hardly any cash, and nobody's like, running their own cards on Square or anything to just take cash out. And I don't count the number of people, but I can sort of see like, how full—" Aria stares at the empty studio, drains her Bakhtini and gives me a steady gaze that tells me that raising her tone at the end of every sentence doesn't necessarily come naturally for her. "I could get really wrapped up in this. I don't want to. I want someone else to worry about it, tell me what's going on, so that I can just love this studio and the people in it. And can I tell you something else?" I nod. She can tell me lots of stuff, particularly if she keeps handing me pink cocktails. Aria puts down her empty glass so that she can put her hands on my mine. "I think I need you here. Your energy. I think you will do more than sort this out."

"I have a package for that." And that is I how I will pay my mortgage, a mantra that will provide no end of comfort as I commit to leaving my dog and my disgruntled spouses for a mat at Yoginitini.

———

The best way to surveil, in general, is from the outside, but this yoga studio is different. Aria told me about the "Gratitude" pouch, the sign-in, the trust, but my domain lies in mapping the terrain between my client's account and the way things actually happen, a frontier I may not glimpse without subjecting myself to the swampcrotch that is group physical exertion.

I always think of these as dog-walking capris, but technically they were designed for yoga (and, maybe, cocktails?) so I pull them on, crate poor, excited Fancy (who, based on the fuss she made when I pointed her toward the crate instead of the leash, also thinks of them as dog-walking capris) and head to Yoginitini.

Considering I know very little about yoga, but a lot about dancing at weddings, "The Funky Pigeon" seems like the right place to start. Now, spreading out my rented mat (two non-expensible dollars in the honor box, no receipt) anxiety sets in. The instructor, Tai, according to the schedule, looks more like a synchronized swimmer than a wedding DJ, especially as she slowly rotates each arm in its socket and twists her torso from side to side.

Even from my spot in the third row, Tai bores into me as we "establish a tunnel of light from the crown of our heads through our sit bones." I wonder what sit bones are. "Rise with me and greet our source!" I recognize that she is introducing us to sun salutations, but, lit as we are by the embers of early evening, the sun is snubbing our efforts. As we stand, lower to the floor and return to standing I recall my experience in a boot camp-style fitness class. The burpee—surely designed as a coping mechanism for a small population so afflicted with the vapors or dipsomania as to need practice picking themselves up off the ground—was treated with such reverence by our solid-looking instructor that I suspected her every sinew was forged in defiance of her debauched and light-headed lifestyle. Tai, by contrast, teaches the sun salutation as if nothing could be more routine than worshiping the exposed industrial ceiling, then dropping in a series of inhales and exhales to the floor. She demonstrates like Ariel, folding and turning into a mermaid, her legs becoming a tail stretched behind her. They flair slowly up and gently settle onto the floor, as slow and silent as if they passed through salt water. My salutation feels neither slow nor silent. After two, my exhales pile on top of each other and dissolve, soft serve dispensed directly into a sweltering palm.

We lunge, we sink from plank, we bring our navels to our spines. I attempt to work out whether the number of knuckles we've been asked to press evenly through exceeds the average for two hands. I lose track.

Tai, klaxon to the maxim, blares: "Inhale abundance! Right foot through and rotate, ankle behind left wrist. And exhale, let go, let pigeon!" Cued by the groans of the lemonites, I anticipate the character-building misery that makes yoga "a spiritual practice." My hips sink, right shin perpendicular to my leg stretching behind me. "Walk your hands. Don't be bullied by the sensation, don't ignore it, recognize it, engage it, welcome it. We hold so much in our hips. Let it go." Eagerly, I wait for sensation to show up. I look around. To my right, a woman sniffles softly into her mat, her head shrugging toward her outstretched arms. To my left, a man winces into his elbows, lips silently mouthing a mantra that, to my trained eye is either "moment's over" or "motherfucker." "Sometimes the only way tension can leave the body is through the eyes!" Tai exhorts when we switch sides. Amid grunts and sighs, I spot released tension leaving trails down my neighbor's cheeks.

I have survived the moments. I have not handed over my lunch money to "the sensation" which sounds like the name of a bully only if your junior high school was also a roller disco. We flop our legs from side to side, then stretch out on our backs, for "this gift of peace and reflection." Given that Tai will not stop talking about the warm light flowing through our joints and muscles and whatnot and how it all flows back to the universe with our breath which is also washing up on the shore and trotting gently like a horse beside the shore, I do not feel super reflective, but I am grateful that class is over. Quothe the pigeon: funk no more. Poe would definitely like savasana.

"Tell me about your practice." I have no idea where Tai came from as I look up from rolling my mat. I have no answer.

"Great class!"

This was not an answer. "Do you do go to Be-You-Tea-Full?" Tai inquires. ShantiShack? Hathahut?"

"Nope, just started here." Tai's face falls briefly, like a film slowed just enough to perceive the darkness between the flash of each image.

Her mouth recomposes itself under empty eyes. "You really need to let the instructor know, you know, if you're new to yoga. I mean, you did very well, your hip flexibility, and your backbeneds . . . someone might push you. You have, a, a SHOCKING amount of potential. Really surprising."

"Thanks. I'm Prana. I'm so sorry, I guess I didn't realize. It just doesn't feel like much to me. I mean, I'm just really focused on telling my left from my right and not falling down." My initial strategy of being just another body in a polyblended sea of integrated shoulder-blades and internally rotated thighs has lasted all of seventy-five minutes.

"Oh. *PRANA*. It's okay. I mean, yes, you clearly struggle with keeping up, and yes, you lack coordination. Clearly. But your inherent *flexibility*. You belong here. I'm Tai. You have very, *very* open hips. I want you to come to my class again."

"Sure. It's great to meet you Tai."

Her eyes don't return my sentiment, but her mouth says "*Namaste*," which I'm pretty sure is Sanskrit for "aloha." Hello and goodbye!

———

I return just in time for a dusk stroll, soft enough light that the good blocks and the bad blocks of East Oakland fade together. In this flattering haze the Fancy recovers from her sulking, reclaiming the dogwalking capris with a definitive schmutz of drool and a streak of hair from a love rub. I limit myself to a cursory tour. I'm thinking about Tai. Something about her inability to conceal her hostility thrills me, and I'm not sure if it's strictly as an investigator. "Not food, Fancy. Not delicious, Fance." Fancy troubles the weeds growing in the cracks after I talk her down from the used condom in the gutter. We putter on, to the broad expanse of lovingly deposited native plants and gardens rolling out before the updated Craftsmen and Victorians of the good block. She looks up at me, bowels still full, as we reach the end of the block. Tai was interested enough to interrogate me about where I practiced, but not so much that she wondered how I paid for the practice I'd just "shared." Not the attitude I'd want from someone working for me, but not exactly stealing either. I slipped a couple bucks in for the mat, but otherwise I didn't even pretend to pay for class. Maybe Tai runs her class on the pusher policy, the first dose is free? My pocket stirs, and I take turn Fancy toward home. "Aria! I was just about to call you. I just got back from Tai's class."

"Wow. 'The Funky Pigeon.'—are you okay? That's a lot of emotional tissue release. Do you need to be alone?"

"Umm, I guess I am alone, sort of." Fancy marches me impatiently toward the corner store, home of the mystery ground treat and everything that could possibly be discarded from a car window. City dog that she is, Fancy loves it all, butts to nuts. "Tai's interesting, I want to take more classes from her."

"You'd love her privates."

"Excuse me?"

"She gives really great one-on-one instruction. Actually, let me see . . . can you come down at 7:30pm tomorrow? She usually has a private lesson before her bartending shifts, but I'm pretty sure her client's still at Bandharoo—Oh my God, you have to follow NorKali on insta, fucking amazing—did you introduce yourself? Will she remember you if I ask her to schedule you for tomorrow?"

I assure Aria that she will and wish her Namaste night. I'm excited. Tomorrow's session will give me the time to inquire about the state of my hips and the stickiness of Tai's fingers. Speaking of sticky, Fancy's dangerously close to the saddest of all street litter, the gutterthong. "Treat! Ooops! Treat!"

Fancy turns, almost smirking. Did she ever intend to put her face in the gutterthong or is she just manipulating a guilty single parent?

"Let me do the investigating from now on, Fance."

Tuesday

I had expected the 10:30 Soulflowin' class to be full of retirees, but instead I see a cornucopia of Bay Area regulars: a clique of nurses; a lithe stringy-haired thirtysomething covered in tribal tattoos and completely hogging the mirror; a lightly goateed woman with close-cropped hair in a wifebeater and bike shorts who helps me gather my blocks and straps; and a middle-aged black guy, sinewy and self-contained. Five signed in, three punched their cards, and one, the narcissist, discretely tucked her twenty-dollar drop-in fee in the pouch. Faryn is completely oblivious to the exchange of lucre on any level. He catches up with the black guy, shows him a new transition that involves breaking up a vinyasa with handstand and then holding both legs at ninety-degree angle from the body. Eventually he notices me and put a surprisingly cool hand on my shoulder.

"Namaste. Welcome. Tell me your name."

"Prana."

His inner body brightens. "That will be so easy to remember. I'm called Faryn. Tell me about your practice, Prana."

"Total beginner."

"Oh." Faryn's eyes dart around the room then lock on mine. Barely audibly, he breathes but mostly mouths "Groupon?"

I follow his lead, cast my gaze around the room, then nod. "Can I hug you Prana?" I nod again. In the middle of a light, not uncomfortable embrace, he whispers, "Prana. This is where you need to be. I can feel a lot of tension inside you and I have to tell you? This place." He backs away, hands still on my shoulders, green-eyes sparkling with bits of amber. "You belong here, Prana. Do what you can, Sweetie. We talk after."

Hugged against my will, made party to meaningful eye contact and forced to hear my own name intoned repeatedly, portentously, and you know what? I love it. I love Faryn. I want to take him around the lake and keep him from eating groundtreats. I never knew it could be like this.

"And now we take it to the second side. Twist and open to the ceiling, let your inner light SHINE." As the long "I" rings out, I see the tremor of jazz hands beginning, but Faryn restrains himself. The slim fit of his short-shorts contrasts with the billow of his tank, which looks stitched together from Stevie Nicks' worn-out stage scarves. I suspect he has to go looser on top so as not to startle us with his wings, our asana angel.

Finally collapsing into my mat, preparing to review the last two hours into my tape recorder once I get back in my car, my list of observations trails off. My head lets the Andean flutes in, and I journey with them, above the tree line, my shoulders melting through the floor, my spine long, my feet unencumbered.

"Gradually get into your body. Are those your fingers? Give a wiggle. Hello toes, can you stop slow dancing and make a little room for the holy ghost? Fantastic! Bring your knees up, hug 'em, love the ones you're with! Let your arms stretch up, and up. Gently roll to your right. Good. Take as much time as you like. We're not here to get fit, we're here to get fetal. Good. Nudge yourself up, you have all the time in the world. Let your head be last, for a change. Yes. Yes. And let's end with an om. In! And! Ahhhhhhhhhhhooooooooooommmmmmmmmm. Beautiful voices from beautiful mouths on beautiful faces with beautiful bodies. It is my privilege to guide you. The light in me salutes the light in you. Namaste."

I roll up my mat as anonymously as I can, pretending to be so centered that I've lost any memory of agreeing to—"Prana! Tell me how you feel. No bullshit, I can't be insulted."

"I don't see why I needed to stick my heel in my anus." Faryn grabs my hand and takes it to his lips.

"I'll buy you a drink and make it up to you. Come by tonight and tell me everything else you hated. I love your energy, it makes me feel really centered."

"Now who's insulted?"

"See? We're already friends."

"See you later."

"No, I see you tonight, Sweetie."

———

Exiting Yoginitini I fall into the warm embrace of Oakland's endless spring. Except it's a little tight, and it doesn't smell like malt liquor. "Prana! You're here!" Aria, still warm and light but too firm for an April breeze, loosens her grip to take me in full. "I almost didn't recognize you, your eyes are so clear, collarbones so broad."

"I can't look so different, I mean you grabbed me pretty fast."

"The basic outlines, sure, but, something's working in you already. I'm so glad that you're—" She sees my finger touch my mouth and then break into sneaky hands (technically, jazz hands straight up and swiftly lowered). Aria seems to catch on, the enthusiasm sneaking out of her tone ". . . so, yeah, welcome, Namaste."

"Namaste." I wonder if it's a coincidence that the sentiment so often comes with a natural shushing motion. Maybe it's also Sanskrit for "please use your inside voices in the library."

I was almost named "Namaste," according to my mother. Totally fascinated by myself and my provenance as only a ten-year-old could be, when Janet Jackson's *Control* album was released I half-convinced her that I should revert back, so I could have a name that sounded like an adjective for the kind of boys with whom Miss Jackson elects to share her marital status. My inability to grasp that "nasty" and "namaste" were different words signifying very different things demonstrates the utter ignorance of my youth. Was there really a moment when I wanted to trade my current annoying Sanskrit name for a different annoying Sanskrit name?

My phone jumps, a text from Aria: "On the dl. Get it! So blessed to have you on the case. Your energy is a gift to our studio." As grateful as I am to have a deep-pocketed, appreciative client like Aria, I'm starting to wish that maybe she could be my mother, too.

I shake the keys in my hand and stroll uphill, to the ever-decreasing strip of non-metered uptown parking. "Hey! Prana!" Faryn waves, then turns on his bike, a Gitane that looks like it has far more coherent memories of the 1980s than Faryn does. He eases it onto the sidewalk next to me, pedaling with the slow drama of a silent film heroine. "You didn't think I was hitting on you before."

I smile. "No, I didn't."

"Bummer. Are you into it?"

This is literally the last thing on my mind.

Faryn doubles down. "It's about energy. And yours, it's so, it's really, like, *man*some, you know? Like in class, the way you were backbending. What depth. And those hips! So open. But still so super uncomfortable. Starting on the wrong side. Almost falling over. It was like watching Matt Damon try to do yoga."

"Should I be flattered?"

"Not beefy Matt Damon, young Matt, gay sociopath Matt Damon! C'mon, just get a drink with me. A warm beverage." Faryn looks at me with utter sincerity and I am stumped. Obviously I should take advantage of every possible opportunity to get to know the teachers. But. I am just straight enough to want a slightly straighter guy to hit on me.

"I really can't right now, my dog—"

"I speak dyke. I get it. You have to wash your hair." Faryn's face falls a little, and it's hard to watch, like Tigger morphing into Eeyore.

"No, I mean, obviously I'm 11/16 gay, but yes, I want to hang out. What's your number?" As he grumbles his number, I compose our first text message: "Tomorrow night (that's dyke for, do you want to get a drink tomorrow night?)? Namaste, Prana."

———

My afternoon return to Yoginitini disrupts the gathering of a rag-tag bunch of lady superheroes. A woman in a strappy tank and the boyshorts embraces a leggy, batik-tighted beauty. Estrogenia and Mandala. Batmandala and Robyn? I'm smiling bigger than I feel. Look at faces, *faces*. Though there was a time when Batmandala's parabolic hindquarters would have inspired me to launch a pro bono investigation; now, broke and aging, her oddly buoyant ass reminds me of how much panty line I must have when I walk the dog. You love me for me, Fancy, but I'm not so sure about the folks strolling behind us.

I no longer expect to derive any meaning from the names of classes. "Shakira's Choice" seems like a great title for a musical about a petite bilingual diva forced to choose a single language for her dance jams. It's a much better icebreaker with the yoga teacher than to go into my clueless yoga-rube spiel again. I turn to the fellow on my right and gesture at Batmandala, "is that our teacher?"

"Nope, you want Michelle, by the foam rollers."

I rise and approach a middle-aged woman in a black sleeveless Obama '08 tee-shirt and striped harem pants. "Are you Michelle?"

"Can you give me a hand with these?" She drapes a dozen black straps across my arms. "No one thinks they need them, but everyone does. Just set one by all the mats in the last couple rows."

"Sure. Umm. So I'm new, I was wondering what this class is for? Maybe I shouldn't be here?"

"Nice to meet you. You're fine. I know, the name's confusing. We relate all our hip-opening stuff back to Shakira, which—I don't know, she's fine but it gives people unrealistic expectations about the music. Welcome."

The rows fill, each mat with an unobtrusive strap nearby. Michelle settles in at the front, forgoing lotus to cross her knees directly in front of her, feet little kickstands at her hips. She sighs heavily. "Let's begin with an om." From the next forty-five minutes she talks us into a bewildering series of poses, somehow convincing me that I should reach under my crotch and hold hands with myself on spread, shaky legs. Rather than demonstrate, Michelle strolls back and forth, sometimes coming down the rows with all the affect of an orchardist surveying a particularly unruly crop of pears. She may be my new favorite.

Finally, she invites us to "explore whatever hip opening challenge you're working on." A man uses his head to pin both legs behind his back. The close, unobstructed view he achieves of his own crotch makes me wonder if any yogi sincerely explains his motivation for increasing his flexibility in mixed company. The Rock would do yoga if he knew about this. "I guess he's not claustrophobic." I mutter. My neighbor smiles back at me guilelessly, without a hint of comprehension, and cups her own lower leg lovingly, like a babe about to be rocked before sliding her shoulder beneath her thigh and popping her leg behind her head.

The instructor, Michelle, smiles at me. "Just relax into cobbler's pose for now. Feel your groin letting go." Let go, groin! I'm surprised to sink farther and farther. Michelle rotates my thighs back and pushes me forward. Startled by her touch, I fart into my own face. My thighs roll back, her knee presses into my spine, and somehow I'm still breathing in through my nose, the gentle compression releasing pressure from less pungent orifices.

Michelle directs us all to lie back. I can just hear her moving purposefully around the room under the sounds of twenty uninhibited respirations. Where is she going? While saluting her light and everyone else's light with my light, I notice that the straps are still out—what errand kept her from sharing our repose? The pouch looks like it just finished its second Thanksgiving dinner and is about to pass out watching the game. What was Michelle up to while we were letting the floor support us, legs rolled away from one another?

———

I swear, if there was some sort of dairy-based rapture sweeping up all the yogurt shops in a column of blue light, the retail space in the Bay Area would shudder and tip like the dishes left behind after yanking a tablecloth. Piedmont Avenue would be nothing but china shards for sure, especially if bubble-tea was called home at the same time.

Fancy's damp, unlicensed but street-smart snout takes us exactly where we need to be: Pilotusize, Piedmont's Premier Pilates and Yoga Center. Technically, this is Oakland, but who am I to articulate arguments against alliteration? At the turn of the century it was a Blockbuster Video. The current iteration retains its octagonal shape, and, crucially, its dedicated parking.

A class seems to just be getting out. I scrutinize a flyer on the window, while Fancy explores the possibility that something delicious might be discovered in her nethers.

"Your friend has great core strength." With her shiny black hair pulled back, Jen's brown eyes and smile seem even broader than usual.

"The world is Fancy's reformer. How now, Jen?"

"Better than you, obviously--are you really interested in the Yin workshop?"

"Which one is that?"

"You get into a pose and hold it for like, ten minutes."

"I could get into that. While we watch those twins from Canada tell people their homes are garbage?"

"No TV, dumbass. Seriously, what's up, Pran?" I'm in luck, catching Jen at her dead hour between lunchtime and "Happening Hour" classes. "Yeah, I wasn't actually going to wipe this shit down anyway." Jen gestures at the rows of machines behind her, identical shiny leather pads on wood with a complicated series of metal springs and nylon straps, each looking like a cross between a medieval torture device and the "intimate furniture" advertised in the back pages of *Maxim* and *GQ*. "You two wanna come in for a sec?"

When we get inside, she gestures to a reformer and takes the one facing it, sliding idly back and forth. Jen makes her sad, caught in the middle eyes until I reassure her that I will not be telling her anything that will make her feel like she's keeping secrets from Iris, her client and friend. "This isn't personal."

"Well, I miss you too!" Jen pouts.

"Oh fuck off! C'mon, you know you can come by whenever, I mean my house is like, eight blocks away from you."

"But those blocks . . . fine, I'm the bad friend. So are you here on business? That's so fancy." Fancy looks up, hoping her name will be followed by the "oops" that means the big hairlesses have made more floortreats! She wags, the angle of her tail forecasting 80 percent chance of treats.

"I'm starting to get into your industry a little."

"Seriously? What yoga instructor files a false claim for workman's comp? Although I guess I could help a lot of people step out on their wifeys . . ."

"Nothing like that. But you've been around a little bit, and I just wanted to feel you out. Yoginitini. Know anyone there?"

"Oh my God, that place is ri-dic-u-lous. Come on? Like anyone should wear yoga pants to a bar? Seriously, it's doing these bitches a favor to make them wear something with a zipper on it at least once a day."

"When was the last time you wore pants that had pockets?"

"This is my job! I'm a Brand Ambassador!" Jen gestures to the logo discretely positioned on the hem of her tank. "Also, I should hide this light under a bushel?" She rises and turns, displaying her magnificent haunches for me, resplendent in purple leggings, then slides forward, sits up again. I am reminded of my original excuse for dating Jen in college: it's not about what she brings to the table, it's what she brings to the *chair*. Jen continues, "Aria's a trip. I mean I hear it's kind of a cool place to work, unless you're looking for a gig that will last more than a couple months."

"Why the turnover?"

"You know, I shouldn't put that on Aria, exactly. I mean, the concept—the studio that turns into a bar at 8:30, it's like, if you teach yoga and you tend bar, you're not necessarily, like, one to stay in a job. I imagine she's pretty attached to her current crew though, if she hired you to spy on them."

"So it seems. But she doesn't have a reputation of being difficult to work for?"

"You work for her, you don't know what it's like?"

"For like, two days. Besides, I'm different."

"Well—" Jen darts her eyes, but her smile tells me it was more for my benefit than her own. She frames her mouth with the back of her hand "she sells two products. One, she knows a lot about, the other, not so much. I mean, she's gone on a lot of retreats and trainings and stuff, but actually practicing with her? Might as well have a podcast and a book. It's a great place to build yourself up. If you were really hungry to make yourself a brand name you get two chances to snuggle up to clients. Then, if you get the right kind of attention, from the right backer. The good teachers just use it as a place to poach students, the bad ones can earn more money bartending somewhere where people wear clothes with buttons."

"Doesn't sound like she knows that much about either product, then." Fancy sniffs and licks a mat, grateful that Jen was thoughtful enough to save a coating of person-salt for her.

"Well, maybe not. Let's just say she's done more shots than Sun Salutations. She's sweet, though, and it's not like Yoginitini's gonna close any time soon. Tons of middle-aged ladies would rather get toasted in their yoga pants and slippers. It's kind of a great concept, really."

"Does she have any competition? Any 'All About Eve's on the horizon? Like Tai, do you know her?"

"Tai. Long limbs, short hair, Oakland booty, vaguely ethnic?"

I nod.

"She's a trip. Hard to know, hot and cold, maybe queer but maybe just needs everyone to wanna fuck her. She used to dance."

"She still could!"

"No, not like that. She was trying to be a ballerina? She was up north somewhere, is there a Seattle Ballet? Anyway, she brings it up enough to sound impressive, but obviously it wasn't for her."

"Because she's . . ."

"Banging, basically. I mean come on, it works in real life, but it's not ballet. She's like one of the 5'7" girls that makes it to the finals of *Top Model*. You've got the skills, the face, but the body—get real! And she's super-competitive, still trying to make it, whatever that means."

"Anyone else you know there?"

"Yeah, there's an older woman, rides the razor between dykey and lazy. Melissa?"

"Michelle?"

"Lots of t-shirt, not enough bra?" I nod emphatically. Jen takes pleasure in monitoring proper ratio of top to foundational garment. "She's been around. I mean obviously, but—have you taken anything from her?"

"Today!"

"Don't hit me, but I can *tell*. You seem so centered, so in your body right now. You're usually pretty loose, but today? Your *prana*'s yoked, stretching toward *dhyana*. Michelle's like, a snake charmer or something."

"Does she have a following? Think she might be building a nest egg, trying to strike out on here own?"

"She definitely has a following, but, shit, takes a lot more than skimming off Yoginitini—but if she wanted the space. It's a fucking amazing space, right?"

"Right, but the weird thing—she's funky around the money, but it goes the *other* way. Would she have any reason to want to keep Aria afloat?"

"You mean, you think they're hooking up?"

"Maybe you could ask around?"

"If you want me to spy you have to pay me, bitch!"

Are we growing apart? I am a little stunned that Jen would tease me about independent contracting. I will soon be buried in IT bills, not to mention the mounting expenses of brining up a rat terrier in this city. "I'll let you know. I'm sorry, how's Lamont?"

"Well, you know labradoodles . . ." Jen's momentary insensitivity fades, a product of the exhaustion brought on by too much time not talking about her dog, my dog, or other people who are young enough, hot enough, or dumb enough to entertain her. I'm surprised Aria didn't at least make the last category, though. ". . . and I'm like, seriously, I am NOT BUY-ING another platypus if you can't leave the stuffing alone for like, a daaay, Lamont!"

"What does Jyn say?" Jen broke a cardinal rule of Sapphic sisterhood by falling in love with someone with basically the same first name, leading to a series of horrific nicknames starting with JJ, J-Fab, J-Fat, J-Chins, J-Chones and gaining complexity throughout their years together.

"Jobama's useless. Keeps giving Lamont pizzles when he doesn't deserve it. Her theory's like, just because he's not grabbing the bull by the horns doesn't mean he can't grab it somewhere else '"

"That's funny—Jyn seemed to disapprove when I bought pizzles for Fancy from her the other day." Ears up, tail a-wag. Am I going to say "oops," Fancy's eyes inquire? What about "breakfast?" Fance is much better at inserting herself into my conversations than I am at attending to more than one mammal at a time. Jen looks at me, expectantly "The pizzle, yeah, Jyn said it wasn't natural."

"Oh, Jay-Z She just thinks it's heterosexist to give pizzles to lady dogs. '99 Pizzles and a Bitch don't get One.'"

Aria was glad to include one-on-one sessions with the instructors at Yoginitini's in my budget, which is the only way I would decide to plunk down $180 for a fifty-minute hour of yoga.

"Praaa-naa. Goooood. Keep your heart ooopen. And. Foooold." Tai straddles me and rests her weight across my back, bringing me face to face with my left knee. I would be tensing up to keep my intestines from announcing that they, too, are open, but that horse left the barn a while ago.

When I heard Tai's rate, I compared it to doms and escorts I've known and judged it a little steep. Now that I see what happens when a beginner—especially a beginner eating her way solo through a CSA subscription built for two—has someone pressing her into shape as she twists and lengthens, it doesn't seem like such a bad deal. I have no idea what you'd have to pay an escort to fart on her, but given the Bay Area's prosperity and diversity, one hundred and eighty bucks is a pretty sweet deal.

She sets a brick between my shoulders and another under my head. "Now fall into the pose. Let your breathing become natural—in through your nose, out through your mouth. Good. Let go of where you've been today. See the frustration, see the perfect version of Prana's day. Let it get bigger and bigger. Now see how it's drifting up. You have the string in your hand. Let go. Let the day that was supposed to be float away. You have everything you need here." A jasmine-scented pillow gently covers my eyes. The studio fills with the gentle sounds of a rustic pan-flute, which doesn't entirely cover the clanking of bottles being moved around, clean glasses set into place, tables and cushions arranged. I have everything I need here.

A few restorative minutes later, I salute the light in Tai and head to the bar. "Try this gin. I'm more of a vodka girl but they distill this in Alameda—I like it with just a hint of cucumber soda." Tai offers me her drink. It opens my heart center. "Want one? I like to throw in a drink with the session, just to give us a chance to check in."

"That's tasty, but I'm afraid I'm a bit of a white wino—I like the hard stuff a little too much to drink it when I'm out."

"Oh, yeah, I get it. I have to be here for a couple more hours, so, you know, I might as well start off right. Dry or sweet?"

"Dry, please."

"Got it." Tai pours half a bottle of La Crema Chardonnay into a glass bulbous enough for the Hulk to stick his pinky akimbo in dainty deference.

"Do you like teaching and bartending, or would you rather stick with one?"

"Yoga's about harmony. I teach that on the mat, I teach that behind the bar. That's my karma. Even with someone like you. You are so naturally gifted in your practice." Tai pauses for a self-effacing response that comes only when I receive compliments I recognize. Tai continues. "I'd much rather teach harmony mixing drinks than teach it by scanning cards and washing towels."

"And not get tips."

"For real! Seriously, this is so much better than working at a gym. Who even goes to a gym anymore?" I try not to look hurt, but I can't help subjecting my arms to a little extra scrutiny as I lift the glass to my lips, subtly flexing my worried bicep.

"Aria seems cool." Could that gin and cucumber concoction be as strong for Tai as it was for me?

Tai smiles and slices citrus, magically keeping her long wavy hair from the cutting board with the flick of a shoulder. "So do you want to know how bad I am?"

Yes. I do, Tai. Tell me everything and forget all the smells I made when you touched me forty minutes ago. "Sorry?"

"Aria has this idea that, like, every drink needs to be about the moment. No premade mixes except tonic water and simple syrup, which, okay, fine. But we're not supposed to prep the garnishes, even. Crazy."

"Is she a tough boss?"

"Oh no, she's great. She's sweet, she's not, not anything like a boss, but you know, I'm not sure how much she went to bars before she opened one, so some of her ideas . . ."

Tai backs away as a group of middle-aged women come in. Purses down on one of the low tables that came out at 8:31 and straight to the bar. "All white wine?" I murmur to Tai, suddenly feeling like we could share a lot of secrets. Tai tilts and gives a short, precise shake, then her face lights up to greet her patrons. "Vodka sodas? I've been infusing this one with almond blossom, you have to try it!"

One of the emissaries sets a generously jeweled hand lightly on my forearm and addresses me. "You were in 'Soulflowin' this morning, right?" I nod. "Your practice, it's obscene." She smiles. "And your backbend—that angle does not exist in nature. Excruciating. I'm so jealous. Have you been studying with Faryn long?"

As I attempt to formulate an appropriately modest response to compliments I'm not sure I comprehend, Tai loads the counter with clear glasses, a single almond blossom floating tastefully amid each cylinder. "We just finished a session. Prana's devotion comes right through, doesn't?"

"Your name is *Prana*? That's lovely."

"Thank you."

Armed with cocktails and a bottle of Pelligrino, she and her friends settle on their meditation cushions and take out Kindles, iPads, and identical paperbacks, marked and ready for discussion. Tai moves to the other end of the bar at the behest of the a man who is allowing his leggings and tank top to define him in areas that I might prefer remain a mystery. I glance at the book club as they compare blossoms. Loneliness sweeps over me in concert with their laughter. I guess this is a real bar after all.

Wednesday

Tracing the classes of your workaday yoga hustler on a map reveals an ideal route for any grey market entrepreneur. All of these women bouncing regularly from the tidy upscale shopping district of Piedmont Avenue to Oakland's hardscrabble downtown to the rapidly gentrifying stretch of San Pablo Avenue that now seems solely occupied by serif-free signs announcing opportunities to practice, to get centered, to flow, to sweat. It's bad enough that I have to try all the classes at Yoginitini—will I have to work the street?

Instead I work the lake. Fancy is not impressed by sun salutations, probably because she doesn't realize how dangerous they are. Yesterday's three and a half hours of inhaling and exhaling through my nose left me sore everywhere else. That pain, and the expertise of my teachers, gives me sufficient discernment to judge the class in progress. A woman's elbows splay out as she sinks into chaturanga, then the she throws her head back, gesturing at a back bend without actually undertaking it. Fancy barks—she knows a cheat when she sees one, but I hustle her along, not so much in fear that Tai will notice me but recognizing that watching people do yoga without being a creep is like patting my head and rubbing my stomach: with practice I could do both, but who has the time? When we stroll back across the grassy, mostly flat area on the side of the lake, the huffing through their noses is over, and the class stretches out, finally breathing through their mouths after in almost a contented, nearly canine repose. You should envy them, Fancy!

Like a slow march of heavy-set slugs, the goose poop gradually colonizes the upper sidewalk. Fancy thinks that means that the odds of dropped sandwiches have suddenly skyrocketed. "What do you have, hmmm? We don't eat that, oh no we don't." For a rat terrier Fancy often looks very sheepish. The sputtering, weak sun seems to be taunting my investment in the 30 SPF face cream, but apparently it's warm enough for these yogis. Amazing how going out in skin-tight clothing with every intention of ending up sighing on your back can get so much support in one context and so little in another. Despite their sartorial courage, Fancy seems as bored with the class as I am. Without music, lights, and whimsical titles, her class isn't terribly invigorating to observe, even if, like me, you're pretending to play with your dog.

I'm lucky Fancy's not that cute. She's almost as nondescript as I am, with my small backpack, short hair, and official East Bay uniform of Oaklandish t-shirt, jeans, and New Balance sneakers. Our other dog, okay, Iris's dog, was the Platonic ideal of Corginess— every trait exaggerated to the extent that he wasn't even Corgi-sized anymore, because that wouldn't allow for the greatest of corgi contrasts, the plump barrel-shaped midsection atop teeny tiny legs, a longshoreman among sherpas, ears aloft, a dog designed by someone who secretly thought Basset Hounds were adorable, but maybe a little tacky, too showy in their floppiness. The Corgi, Orpheus G. Freidman, was a local legend, adored by the residents of the group homes and retirement homes alike. Danny Glover, whom Iris assumed was just an extraordinarily handsome older black guy, caught Orpheus's smile and froze in his tracks. "You're a star, fella. That's right!"

I suppose there's a cruel irony in naming this completely loyal, perfectly dog-like rat terrier "Fancy" in Orpheus's shadow, but who can resist the opportunity to write "Fancy Freiberg" on every form? Little did I know that writing down your dog's full name is generally the first step in a very expensive, if not traumatic process. The innocence of my unencumbered self makes me pity her, until I remember her pristine furniture and hairless linen and I start to hate her just a little.

——

Seventeen variations on forward folds later, class is Namastely over. Tai shakes herself like a damp Fancy and settles into lotus until a paper bag, casually tossed by a fitness walker lands at her feet. She doesn't look inside, brings it to her heart chakra. Tai mounts a road bike, backpack and mat cross on her back, and she's gone.

Fancy and I get up to complete our circuit around the lake and catch up to our fitness walker. "Not food for you, Fancy!" Why do people bring stale bread for these monsters, enable the squatting of ungrateful waterfowl? Not only is it giving encouragement to evolution's greatest slackers, but some of us have gluten-free dogs. "You like that Fancy, but you don't like your eczema. Come on, come on!" Fitness walker is spry as hell but does a good job hiding her hurry, her now-empty hands butchering the air with the such regularity and aplomb I half expect to see her in a bloody apron, should she turn around. Which she won't. Because she's. Going. Too fast.

——

We have lost our fitness walker.

We continue around the lake, positioned, as we are, almost directly opposite my car. As Fancy turns me around—"And now we go this way"—I see the patch of grass formerly covered with blankets and mats is now occupied by a boot camp.

I turn Fancy back around, now purely for the scenery, the walk. The scent of bird poop, the unwelcoming odor of second-hand fish hangs over the southeast corner of the lake like a Pashmina on a Olsen twin. Why don't I live here? Even this side of the lake would be better. "Come, Fancy." Fancy likes our yard, but she could do with less, for sure, and I could do without the drug deals and casual hold-ups. I'm better, I don't shudder or bite my lip anymore, but every time I answer my phone I'm reminded that it's not the one I wanted, it's just the one that wasn't taken by the teenager who accosted me at 8am on my way to the bus stop. Lips meet teeth. I guess I'm not feeling as over it as I thought.

"Purr-eye-a-vet ice! They're wa-tchin you!" Okay, ringer off in public, got it.

"Weinberg investigations."

"Is this Prana? I need to speak with Prana Weinberg."

"This is Prana."

"So, like, I never, nee-ver, never would consider doing anything, like, I guess shady?"

"Who is this?"

"Yeah, so that's not—that's not super-crucial?" I glance at the number again. No name or city came up, thought it was 415 but it's 425—not San Francisco or Marin, but Washington, Seattle area.

"Okay."

"Yeah, all you need to know is, DUCK!" That's the pop that's not a car, not Chinese New Year, and Fancy knows it's not. Down, down from the path, to the low tide retaining wall. Is this really where I want to be? Did I slide down here?

"Hey, you're fine. And you'll be fine. But Yoginitini's? Not fine, and just, like, let them be not fine, kay?" Tires squeal—I hear it on the call and I hear it in my other ear. Is he in the car? I should keep him on the line.

"Hey, can I do anything to clear this up?" I listen for wind on the line, for something to tell me if he's still at the park.

"Find another studio." That's the beep. Was he in the car? I scroll back into my phone and listen to see if I can hear any difference in quality from the beginning to the end. I definitely have the bay wind, then—but then some of the noise is from my side too.

"C'mere Fancy." We'll just stay. I'll try to keep my lips together, teeth apart and breath until I feel like it's worth the risk.

"No dogs. No dogs on the beach!" Or we'll stay until bossy Asian lady kicks us out. That's fine too.

———

As soon as we reach the street level, my right hand shudders—I'm still white knuckling my phone, a wanted woman. I take Fancy beneath me, hit the deck. Can the shooter really still be here? They can't be in a car—a window, one of the condos? In through the nose, I can hear it in Michelle's voice now. The phone jumps again in my hand.

"Whattayouwantfromme!"

"Umm . . . yeah so, it's been live for a couple days now? Any issues?"

"Jesus. Josh. Hey."

"Is this, is this not a good time?"

"No, no, this is perfect. Are you at your office?"

"Upstairs. Come by."

"Would it . . ."

"S'not a consult, Prana. Following up's'all. Just come by, I'll buy you a coffee. Or maybe a chai? You sound pretty wired already."

"See you in ten."

Fancy knows the way to Farley's, though she seems pretty convinced that it would be shorter going the other way around the lake. Some kind of canine radar tells her where all the Oaklanders too clumsy to eat and walk at the same time congregate each day, a surf report for the culinarily adventurous canine. Fancy heads decisively toward 20th as I try to point her at Grand, but she's determined, certain that somewhere on Lakeshore there's a hunk of burrito ahead that the ants and the birds don't know about yet. "Later, Fancy. I need you to guard me right now."

———

I trust Fancy to the eager clutches of the Berkeley students outside and ascend to Farley's loft, carefully avoiding the politely dazed crowd fiddling with the magazines while awaiting their snacks and beverages. Josh pushes his stool back from the counter overlooking the street and awkwardly embraces me.

Oh, right. I must look really horrible right now. I don't realize how scared I've been until I feel myself fighting the urge to sink into his arms, to transfer all my weight to his delicately pot-bellied frame. I resist. Josh smells a little like balls. Also, I'm sad that my IT guy thinks I look like I need a hug. I need a hug. Maybe I should have gone to SoulFlowin' with Faryn this morning. He hasn't texted me back about tonight, which is a shame because, fuck it, going out for a drink tonight might start right now.

"I think I see Fancy down there. 'Sup Fancy?" Fancy does not hear Josh's greeting, nor does she recognize "sup" as a salutation, but I respect his ability to recognize my partner.

"Yeah, let's head down." I think I need something cold.

"CoolyeahIneedarefill." I think of the airflow produced by Josh's avid wave to Fancy, moments earlier, and judge, silently, that he has probably had enough coffee for 3:30pm. Josh sets up a blockade of purpose-made gear bags and an outdated Cook's Illustrated to hold his spot, tucks his laptop into his messenger bag, and ushers me down the stairs, empty mug in hand. The wholesome biracial girl with what looks like stubby wine corks through each earlobe takes his mug from him and gets to work on my order, a simple one for a coffee shop. White wine. Whatever is three dollars at happy hour. Please. She hands over a rocks glass too full for my shaky hands. She is my hero.

"Yeah, so what's up?"

"There were gunshots at the lake."

"Right."

"No, but these, I think these were actually for me."

"Whoa, what, how would you . . ."

"I got a call while it was going on, they said they could see me and to lay off."

"Lemme see your phone." Josh is wired, looking at my phone like Fancy looks at her leash after a day in the crate.

"I can't really afford—"

"Don't worry about it, I wanna see . . ."

Josh listens to my story with slightly more interest than Fancy, who's distracted by our proximity to that whimsical sandwich place where everyone eats off an ironing board. They're famous for their chicken, but in Fancy's mind it's the no-room-for-error dining surfaces that steal the show. That, not the locally sourced bread, is her chicken-delivery-system.

I fill Josh in on our run-in at the lake, judiciously tugging at Fancy's leash whenever she gets a little too close to the rash-delivery systems cunningly protecting the chicken. I can give Josh just enough of my attention to explain Tai's lakeside delivery. "What did this, package, what did it look like?"

"It looked . . . like that!" Josh follows my eyes.

"Was it a sandwich?"

"Well, I don't know, but what about the bullets, the warning?"

"See your phone again?"

"Here." I take a deep drag off second-hand smoke from a squatting bike messenger. It's a tease.

"I mean, the number's right there."

"Seriously? I have an investigator's license. I know how to get incoming numbers off my phone."

"No I know, I just—lemme think if there's anything, anyone I know that can help figure out who called."

My wine is broken. It was sitting right in front of me, working just great, and now it is all gone. "You know what? I'm not mad at you, I'm mad at myself. I think I figured out what Tai had delivered."

"What?"

"A sandwich."

Fancy's antsy. Literally. She is racing with ants to a discarded roll. "I should go. Clearly it's someone's d-i-n-n-e-r time."

"Dinner time?" And Fancy's off. I wave to Josh and hold up my phone. We'll talk soon. Now how will I tell Aria that one her instructors is secretly . . . eating gluten?

———

"Hello Fancy! Hello . . ." Iris's doorman looks genuinely apologetic as he forgets my name. I sympathize, though I not only remember his name but also his preference for those who forget it to refer to him as the "doorman" rather than employing the neutral "door operator." Fair enough. After investing untold time, psychic energy, and money, Rafa has a proud thin mustache produced from a stock of relatively recently acquired testosterone. In true bay area fashion, when I originally asked about his name at the beginning of Fancy's joint tenure as a child of divorce, he claimed total ignorance of the glory and career of Rafael Nadal, whom he resembles, with his inky hair side-parted and shellacked and his studiously flat chest puffed, not a bit. I'd feel bad putting Rafa in the middle of our custody woes, but for my notion that he likes to have extra cause to chat with Iris. I can't blame him for that. He tries to find my name again. "How's it going . . ."

"Not Fancy. I'm Fancy's friend with the good personality. Prana. It's okay, I know which of us is the pretty one. Is she in?"

"Hey, Fancy's family. She's always welcome."

"Right, and you probably shouldn't say about . . ."

"Nah, don't worry about it." Rafa brushes the crumbs from Fancy's maw. "You look a little sleepy. Mama take you all the way around the lake?" He looks up again flashing the broad smile of a former dog-crazed tomboy. "So, see you Friday?"

"Yeah, will you be here?"

"Sure, after ten. In fact, That'd be a great time, actually anytime between 10 and 8."

"I'll be here."

———

I've dropped off my dog, I have vague-ish plans with a hot gay yoga instructor (wrong kind of gay maybe, but still), my car's on that secret strip of Harrison where I can leave it until the streets are cleaned on Tuesday morning, and I haven't heard nearby gunshots for hours. Why do I just want to go back to work?

And work comes back to me. I see Michelle walking purposefully toward up Telegraph, weaving through the crowd with a rollie suitcase and a hatbox. Now I know why she looks so familiar to me. I paint over my image of Michelle from the studio with generous, sparkly red lips, powder-porcelain cheeks, eyes highlighted and circled like the vocab words from last night's homework. Michelle is Chica Boom, and she's got a show at the Stork Club tonight.

Once I'm inside, I sink into a booth like a warm bath. I've been putting off updating Aria, but I send her a text with a promise I can mostly deliver: "Meet Friday? I have news!" Surrounded by PBR-swilling kids, drinking an over-strong vodka tonic, parked at the "reserved" table near stage right, I feel observed, but in a way that makes me feel safer than I've felt since the shots at the park. I'm only allowed this seat because the painted, generously bosomed women instinctively made room for me, as royal consort of the famous Iris Isersmilink. I didn't have to wear a camera or give anyone a bump. Iris is discrete, clearly she's only told her inner circle about the break-up. But these dedicated fans, while they know her signature swipe of lipstick, applied from her cleavage-encased tube to her lips, and they've seen the way her legs emerge, swan-like from a carefully maneuvered cascade of feathers, they never even knew my name, and now they feel closer to her, sitting with me.

The rest of the audience, rambunctious in a collective cry for discipline, sits on the Stork's beer-glazed floor. "You are not over the hump. This is 'Boom,' ladies and jerks! This is the top of the hump." The emcee, Dali Farton, helpfully mimes what one might accomplish at the top of a hump, then explains how burlesque works to the newbies with the help of her fans. " 'Boom''s pretty high-falutin, but I like to be comfortable. The thing is, as comfortable as this housedress is . . . when . . . it . . . gets . . . loud . . . and the music—oh no!" Her dress is on the floor, revealing carefully coordinated y-front manties, suspenders, and a tank. The screaming continues and I scream along, not because I needed to see Dali Farton in her undies but because I finally realize how much I need to scream, dogless, haunted, shot at.

"That's right, get your generosity on y'all, it's interignition!"

Performers crowd the stage, looking both exposed and covered by virtue of their old-timey underthings. Nothing is worse than old panties in an intimate moment, but here in public they generate throaty hoots. They come for us, seeking our generosity on every side, negotiating the bodies that cover the floor with surprising ease, the way an elephant can seem bored descending a steep riverbank. All in a day's work. As the girls pass, I can see Michelle, her hat filling with sticky one-dollar-bills. Is this the unlikely pouch bulge Aria's so worried about? My phone jumps. "Where are we going?" Faryn texts.

Dali holds the mic a little ways from her face so that she can really holler: "And after the show, it's the?"

"AFTER PARTY" the crowd shouts back. We're not dummies. We even know what comes after the hotel lobby. I ease myself through the packed bodies to get another drink. I aim my shoulder down and make it around the line for PBR tallboys, only to square up to the bar behind a familiar behind.

She turns, perfectly made-up but for her bare-look lips that will still leave a moist outline on her rocks glass. "Iris! Hey."

"Hey" Iris says, pivots right, and disappears backstage.

I want to hear "Don't You Forget About Me." I want to see Iris her dip her head to apply her tit-mounted red lipstick while I cheer, a bubble among a sea of hoots and screams. More than watching her number, I want to hear her demure, later, that if people knew how easy her tricks were they wouldn't cheer, that the real trick is keeping glitter off the sheets.

I turn left and leave the bar.

As the air hits me I find myself gulping at it like I'm coming up from a dive. The sudden visceral hunger reminds me of the gluten-free vegan brownie my table-mates forced on me.

"Kim's" I text Faryn, the brownie already nestling itself in my stomach.

———

Kim acknowledges me with a snort and goes back to her newspaper, scanning up and down columns of text that, for all I know, might be reporting the latest speculation about the true contents or provenance of a celebrity "baby bump," but given the satisfied grunts emanating from the reader, I suspect it's about money. I head directly for the jukebox. I put on Earth Wind and Fire. Before I can settle into my favorite booth, Tammy strides past from the patio. She knows my whistle's for her and turns, lighter and pack of American Spirits stashed in a granny-style leather wallet in one hand, dregs of a greyhound lazing about in a sweaty tumbler gripped in her right, which she sets down at my table hard enough that the last few sips nearly escape.

"Hot date?"

Tammy sighs. "Welcome to the afterparty. My single black male in tech turned out to be a data entry clerk."

"Total stoner?"

"Hugging him was like driving over a skunk. Not compatible with my lifestyle as a motherfucking public safety officer." Tammy tilts her head back, pouring the remnants of her drink down her throat. "Where's your drink?"

"I think I'm meeting someone."

"I think I know who." Tammy jerks her head toward the door where Faryn, be-scarfed in a loose tank over leggings printed with butterfly wings, scans the bar. His eyes find mine. He flicks both ends of his diaphanous scarf with the backs of his hands as if pushing through saloon doors and presents himself to Tammy.

"Faryn. Delighted."

"Tammy. Thirsty. Am I playing this right?"

"Prana. Also thirsty. Why don't you two sit and I'll get us something to drink?"

The floor feels soft, each step feeling as if it should be accompanied by the burp of broken suction. The bar never gets any closer, like a water tower on an Iowa byway. "You drink?" My reverie broken, I nod at Kim, hold up the number three, slap down a twenty, and am grateful that the consistency of my bad habits enables their frictionless indulgence. Faryn grabs two of the greyhounds and eyes me strangely. "Are you okay?" It takes all my concentration to keep my drink level while I slide back into the booth. Faryn's still looking at me. It feels like everyone at Kim's is looking at me. The greyhound tastes strangely sour. I remember my brownie. I remember why I may have forgotten my brownie.

"Holy shit. I'm stoned." Tammy looks disgusted. "I had a brownie at the show, Iris was there, I was confused. It was vegan and gluten-free and—"

"Full of THC. Seriously, how am I supposed to be a cop and have a social life in this town? Fuck me." Faryn leans in toward Tammy.

"You're a cop?"

"Enough that I don't eat the baked goods that they sell on the street."

"Interesting." Faryn, more than politely, prods Tammy through her whole story, which Tammy reveals with the polish and cheer of someone who's already sailed through tech and dress, ready for the bright lights. As if taking Tammy's cue, the whole bar seems brighter. I can feel my pupils struggle to adjust, and finally they lose patience with the whole endeavor, going to break without clocking out.

Thursday

"They're watching you watching you watching you ooo-ooo."
I don't feel good enough to be my secretary. And this is not my couch. I send it to voicemail, wishing the throbbing in my head was as easily dismissed by swiping left.

"Is that Prana? On my davenport?" Faryn sets a coffee down on the table in front of what might be the world's least comfortable white leather couch. "Scooch!" Sitting up gives the blood in my head a place to go. "You said your car would be okay overnight, but I thought maybe it was all a ruse. Then you passed out."

"Where?"

"14th and Madison." A mental picture forms of the other side of this light-filled studio.

"Nice place."

"Bought *early*, when people still thought Lake Merritt only had one good side. Drink up, Prana. Caffeinate and all is coming."

"Thank you. I'm so, so sorry. I know what happened, but fuck. Even on a good night I'd be a shitty date, but last night . . ."

"If I thought someone was shooting at me, I know I'd get messy. Though, to be fair, no one *has* to shoot *at* you to get shot. I only really notice how bad it is when my folks come to visit. Of course, I'm not *Prana Weinberg, MA PHR PI*! You must be in gunfights all the time! You should be on TV!" My reflexes are so dulled I can't feel my eyebrows shoot up. I shared so much more with Faryn than his excessively bright apartment last night.

"I should get out of your hair—or, can I get you breakfast or something?"

"You don't remember last night at all, do you?"

There are five stages of Prana stoned in public. Stage one: I am high! Stage two: Everyone is high! Stage three: Everyone is better at being high than I am! Stage four: I am maybe better at being high and drunk! Stage five: I am maybe not so good at making sure a surface is free from food items or electronic devices before I lie down!

"I have a pretty good idea."

"Uhmm, well, it's almost 10:30. We're meeting Tammy at that place with the pork buns that's only open 11:15 to 2. We won't get a counter spot at this rate. Move it!"

"It's not Michelle. Absolutely not." Faryn fairly skips down Harrison.

"I am never eating anything at a burlesque show again."

"Are you hungover?"

"No I just can't believe, I mean, I can keep secrets. I was a human resource manager—I knew about peoples' DUIs and shit. I can't believe I told you everything. I should quit."

"No. Aria's just going to hire someone else. We need you!"

"We'll see." It occurs to me that there's very little reason to be any more forthcoming about the case than I have already. "Do you teach anywhere else?"

"No time. I do privates here and in the city, plus modeling—can't believe I'm going for pork buns!"

All that flows from Faryn's mouth for the next ninety minutes will just as easily seem like a series of double-entendres or euphemisms for varsity-level sex acts. Tammy and I don't mind at all. In fact, Tammy seems ready to multiply every *entendre* she can draw from Faryn's *bouche* when he takes his leave, thanking Tammy for "getting me up in these buns!"

As Tammy takes me back to Zsa Zsa, I make a final attempt to recover information, if not dignity from my misspent evening. "So you and Faryn . . . hit it off?"

"I know. It's weird, and it was your date, but come on! You two would be hopeless trying to be straight together."

"Right, well, he might not be my type, exactly." Tammy's snort sounds almost painful, as if she's shifted the contents of her sinuses violently enough to trigger an airbag. "What? I thought you were on the hunt for someone with a real job."

"He doesn't *need* a real job. Weren't you listening last night? He owns a building in the Marina. Oh shit, tell me everything about his place, I couldn't figure out a way to invite myself to put you to bed there last night. This is you."

"Not me. It's extremely bright. I mean, it's nice, I don't know. Not me."

"But you do drive a car that looks just like that."

"Yeah, but it's the gold one we want, it's past the Whole Foods. No, that's a Camry."

"Y'all act like you can't tell brown people apart. 'That's a Camry.' This is it. Your Honda Accord."

"One of them. Thanks Tammy. Let's hang out."

"Definitely. I want to go to yoga with you."

"Jesus." Tammy blows me a kiss and disappears up the hill, visions of low sexual expectations and high bar tabs dancing in her head.

———

I have just enough time before Tai's class to do a little research. Like SCUBA-diving and cornrows for white people, yoga requires a "journey." To this journey add at least one of the following: a sports injury: some sort of personal or family illness, including but not limited to childbirth; an encounter or series of encounters with a long list of unfamiliar names, each of whom is credited with catalyzing to revelation of a heretofore unknown authentic self. To my disappointment, even Faryn's bio on the Yoginitini website follows the template:

> The severed ACL that ended Faryn's basketball career was the catalyst for a mind-body journey with no end in sight. His physical therapist recommended hatha yoga as a way to cope with the lingering tightness and asymmetries from decades of abusing his instrument as if it were merely a ball-delivery device. Since then, Faryn has studied with Rukishri Deva, Jasmine Savage, Franklin Folder, and Justina Adaré, among other. When he shares his practice, he strives to be a joyful vessel so that the wisdom of his body inspires his students to seek wisdom in their own.

None of their bios mention a history of larceny or threatening well-meaning investigators with firearms. Still connections to the suburbs of Seattle, Washington, also known as the 425 emerge:

> Michelle's interest in sonic healing led her to Bellevue, where she earned a 300 hour certification in BioSonic Wellness Coaching. When not teaching or practicing, she bring ease and light by playing her didgeridoo at farmer's markets, festivals, and rituals throughout the Bay.

Iris always said, a healer's a healer, whatever they do. Jen never explained what she meant when she said Michelle's class brightened my prana's yolk, but I definitely felt something. Not enough to listen to a didgeridoo, but something. Tai's bio simply says, "Tai combines the discipline forged from her years with Pacific Northwest Ballet with her lifetime as a seeker to make every class an opportunity for transcendence." Another potential denizen of the 425, though less direct, since there's no evidence that she lived in the Seattle suburbs. Still, it seems pretty important to be on time for Tai's 10am "AB-BUN-DANCE Flow" class.

———

Magda, the creamiest of the fleet, brushes her lips against the Prius in front of her as she squares her tail before the Prius behind her. I whisper my apologies as I sprint down Grand Avenue, turn on Telegraph, and make it to Yoginitini just in time for Tai's welcome.

"Shake it out. Like you mean it. Side to side. Hands up and scream it! What's our dream?"

"Abundance?"

"What's our dream?"

"Abundance!"

"We manifest?"

"ABUNDANCE!"

"Climb, and shake. Climb, and shake. Now shout out to the sun, bring it down!" I'm relieved that "shout to the sun" apparently means the exact same thing as a sun salutation except we're trying to pull through into upward facing dog to the throbbing beat of Yanni mixed by Major Lazer.

Tai finally takes us to the floor. The exhaustion brings out my animal nature. I fight the urge to circle my mat on my hands and knees and then lie back, belly ready for a scratch. "ZiiiiiiiiiiIP. Navel to your spine. And lift, and roll." I try to raise and lower my vertebrae individually, as instructed. Is this what Tai means by "zipping up my midline?" If I were Amish, would I have to imagine a series of hooks and loops?

"Bring your knees to your chest. Embrace. Accept. Squeeze like it's the last day of retreat. And let them go, thighs roll away from each other, palms open to the fading light. SHAAAA-va-sanaaaaaaaaaaah." Wales or dolphins send messages of love across the depths, the gentle rustle of the tambourine setting the beat. The man next to me snorts, the sputters of his cardiovascular system shifting into neutral. Tuning in, beyond my neighbor's deviated septum I hear the light padding of bare feet across the floor. I open my eyes. Tai stares into them from across the room. I close my eyes. Fuck.

I was safe during the final Namaste round. Like dodging the path of a sprinkler, my position in the middle of the studio misses the spray of gratitude. Head up, stage right, penetrating gaze, hands together and Namaste, head humbly lowers comes around and raises, returning to its highest point at the far left side of the arc, hands still on the forehead. Still, it takes everything I have to spray and wipe down the rental mat instead of bolting for the door. Each stroke turns into a careful spiral scrub. I will my eyes to follow the path of my wash cloth rather than meet Tai's gaze, currently boring a hole through the back of my head. Yet when I've finally massacred every bacterial settler on this scrap of PVC prairie, Tai is gone.

Hustling north on Telegraph to Magda, a familiar scarf flares in my peripheral vision as I pass twenty-fourth street. I cross Telegraph and cross back, this time approaching the intersection with more care, phone set to absorb any conversation that might seep my way from twenty-fourth. Adopting the weary gait of someone who went much lower in chair pose than I ever have, I see Tai, draped in a very Faryn-esque scarf, in some sort of intense conference with a swarthy fellow, mostly obscured his phone but clearly conducting more business than he can handle at once, if Tai's gestures are any indication. I linger just ahead of them on Telegraph, staring at my phone with all the intensity that I'm putting into listening to their exchange. My ears squint with the strain, but after ninety seconds, as much time as anyone over thirty can be expected to stop on the street and play on their phone, I resume my march to Magda.

———

In my audio lab, which, to the untrained eye, looks like a silver late-model Honda Accord, I scrutinize the results of my snooping. I play with the levels, turning up each frequency in turn. While I never find a setting that reveals an admission of guilt from, I do have what sounds like Tai, inquiring, "Am I gonna have to slice that mustache off your assface, assface?" At least I was reading her body language correctly. I turn over the engine and take the audio lab a few blocks up the street to see if Jen has any insight into the mustache's possible owner, and whether "assface" means that the mustache in question might be vertical rather than horizontal.

"Neighbor!"

"Whatever" Jen says back, giving me quick hug while Jyn restrains a very agitated Lamont. She takes me past her life partners, grabs two glasses, plucks a pink bottle from the fridge, and wedges the sliding door open with an elbow. "You always show up at wine o'clock," she says as she gestures to a patio chair. She fills two glasses

"On the dot!" I lean forward and our glasses meet.

"So how's 'Prana Weinberg and the Lost Yoga Revenue?'"

"A little frightened, actually." Jen refills my glass as I recount my misadventures at the lake. Faryn knows everything, so I need to nail this down, like, yesterday, because he doesn't seem like someone who can keep a secret."

"Right. Plus, how do you know Faryn's not the thief? You said it sounded like a dude on the phone threatening you the other day"

"Not just threatening me—bullets, Jen! Bullets at me and Fancy!"

Jen's mouth shuts and stretches, her eyes begin to bulge. "Jen?"

"Sorry." She coughs, straightens up. "Can't, hic, listen and drink at the same time." I return to my glass of wine as she settles herself. "Am I a horrible person that I think it's hilarious that anyone would do a drive-by to thwart an investigation into a yoga studio?"

"It's not hilarious, it's just Oakland."

"Fine, okay, so some guy called, but it's not Faryn because you didn't find a gun during your careful recon mission in his apartment last night?"

"Fuck you. No, the voice was definitely not Faryn. It was, like, self-consciously deep, not Faryn's voice at all. But, it *was* familiar. I don't know."

"And the area code was 425? If someone at Lake Merritt's going to take a shot at you—"

"AND FANCY!"

"Fancy was there, too, of course. I just, I mean, have you been to the Seattle area? Bellevue? Redmond? There's like, Microsoft, horse trails, and Indian buffets, and, well, it's not very, um, agro, if you know what I mean. I was in Bellevue for a couple weeks for those Eflorescent™ color therapy workshops. Oh my god. Such healthy, homely people. Not a single person, male or female, wearing pants that they couldn't go climbing in. Jeez-uz. And I was like" Jen jerks her head toward Jyn, trimming Lamont's nails just inside the sliding glass door, "please, don't let the Dog Whisperer ever visit and get ideas. They will wear fleece vests to their own fucking weddings up there!" Jen's disquisition on the unisex stylings of the Pacific Northwest provides more comfort than insight.

"Your disquisition on the unisex stylings of—"

"Okay, okay, I just think, if the limbs zip-off, don't wear it to tapas. Or sushi. Coffee, okay, maybe brunch, but—"

"You wear work-out stuff . . . "

"But it *fits*! And it's nice!"

"Fine. So you don't think Fancy and I are in danger because we're being threatened by someone who's probably got a roomy crotch-gusset. You're right. I feel so much better." Jen refills my glass. My annoyance with her is inversely proportional to the level of rosé in my glass.

"Chin up, sister. You pick up Fancy tomorrow and you go back to serving papers if you want. You're not a Hardy Boy. Fancy does look kinda like Angela Lansbury, though."

Friday

I sleep late, at least for me. I am a victim of too much rosé and not enough small dog to drag me outside for a 6am constitutional. My yoga clothes smell stale and lightly acidic, a combination of yesterday's vigorous practice and fermented grapes. I wedge the girls into yesterday's bra and today's panties, convince myself that my leggings are just cold, not damp, pull them on, and grab my keys. Outside I hold them up and see which headlights flash as I remote unlock, a practice Iris was pretty sure would on day invite a car-jacking, but makes me feel like Batman. Zsa Zsa blinks hard, and I sprint toward her fool's beige embrace.

I take the last spot in the class, directly before Michelle, who seems pretty preoccupied with a tiny notebook covered in a fabric reminiscent of the Guatemalan harem pants I used to leaven the solemnity of my Sub-Pop t-shirts in the early nineties. She glances as my mat snaps loudly into place, then goes back to her book. "Huh. Okay." Michelle lets her head fall to the left, then the right, but doesn't invite us to follow her. "You are clear!" Michelle's eyes are closed, book left open beside her. She continues:

"O rose, cut in rock,
hard as the descent of hail.

"I could scrape the colour
from the petals
like spilt dye from a rock.
If I could break you
I could break a tree.

"If I could stir
I could break a tree—
I could break you."

We listen to ourselves breathing, the cogs working out the inspirational tone nearly audible. Still listening. Just when I'm about to wrench my neck for a peek at the clock, Michelle begins. "Stand at the top of your mat. And inhale hands UP!" Michelle talks us through two sun salutations, then brings us down to our mats. "Jump through, press into your palms, *dandasana*, and fold. *Paschimotanassana*. Tails up, navel in, press your legs into the floor, if you bind, bind." After tilting my pelvis and driving into my sit bones and leading with my sternum, she has us watch as she transforms herself from sloppy middle-aged lady to ninja. "Start on your back, tuck the right heel, left leg out. Pop up!" Michelle regards us with brutal indifference as she takes warrior one, tucks, switches her legs and rolls back up into warrior one on the other side. "I'll give you somewhere to start, but this is where you're going." Just switching my legs on each roll takes a level of concentration I generally associate with parallel parking or *BuzzFeed* quizzes revealing which *Veronica Mars* character should be my co-parent. "Use your hands. Then let the weight come out of your hands." I plant into the front leg and push into the back, making wobbly warriors left and right, my hands getting lighter and lighter. "Not bad. The next time you come up on your right, hold it. Hold it. Lean forward. Reach and lift your back leg." I'm falling on my face I'm falling on I'm

———

Michelle plays Joan as Policewoman. I try to reconcile my rudimentary understanding of gravity with the incontrovertible proof, thanks to warrior three, that falling on your face while sober is more challenging than almost any yoga posture. How many warriors are there? Why are my inhalations so much easier to lengthen than my exhalations? Who smells like balls?

"Stretch. Rotate. Shake if you want. Squeeze your knees and roll up, one last time. Sit. Don't look at me. Look at each other." I meet the eyes of my fellow students. You, small fellow with the mustache in the ribbed white tank. You smell like balls. "Namaste."

I take my time wiping off my mat, enjoying the post-yoga atmosphere.

"But, is it yoga?" Batmandala asks her neighbor as she returns her hair to its pre-inversion bun.

Robyn assures her. "Everything Michelle does is yoga." Currently Michelle's yoga includes taking a large quantity of one-dollar bills and exchanging them for a much smaller quantity of fives and twenties. Mystery solved. Apparently my yoga for today will include a visit with Aria Butler, likely accompanied by a certain rat terrier-about-town.

———

As I return to Zsa Zsa, I'm summoned. Tammy's text says, "Let's talk. Can you come by ASAP?"

"Now? Coated in yoga stank."

Sometimes I forget the conditions of Tammy's labor. She calls. "Prana, what part of 'our canine unit is incontinent' do you not understand? Get down here."

A few minutes later, and I'm downtown, and not the only one marinating in their own juices. Still, I'm white and fit enough to have a relatively easy time getting to the Office of the Inspector General, Tammy's domain, and the closet where she reviews approved acquisitions requests, monitors compliance with the negotiated settlement, and maintains a tumblr devoted to matching screen grabs from *The Real Housewives of Atlanta* to Maya Angelou quotations. I'm honored that she had time for the likes of me.

"Thank God! Prana. Look." One of her monitors displays a black and white photo of Nene Leakes, mouth too full of venom to completely close. Tammy has tastefully placed in script near the bottom the Angelou quote, "There is no greater agony than bearing an untold story inside you."

"Too obvious? Tell me."

"This is why I had to park in a garage downtown? To help with your tumblr?"

"Of course not. No. I put out some feelers on that shooting."

"Thank God. I'm supposed to pick up Fancy today, but, fuck, if I'm making her a, a target! I just. I couldn't live with myself."

"Yeah, I think Iris might not like it either. Oh right, she can't live with you anyway. Did I tell you, Faryn and I are going to Kabuki Springs Tuesday? It's unisex day, so everyone will be in swimsuits, but still. Mike would never, ever—"

"My dog. My person. Physical safety. Can we get back to that, please?"

"Fine. So first of all, I can't believe you didn't check this out."

Tammy gestures to a map of the lake, laden with pictograms—needles, fists, cars with wavy lines behind them, clearly representing crimes reported in the last week at each point on the map. She points her cursor at an image of a revolver on the southeast end of the lake. A familiar date pops up. "I know there were shots fired then. I was there."

"But watch this." Tammy does a history progression. Time runs backward on the map as robberies, assaults and public disturbances move around the lake, disappearing popping up, clustering, unclustering. The still center is the white revolver on a field of purple, flashing but static. "I just don't think you should take that so personally, you know?"

"That's a lot of shots in one place." I raise my voice "you'd think the police would be interested in an observation like that."

"Oh, fuck off, you know that's not my job. Here's the deal: pretty heavy concentration of fire-cracker-happy households plus very paranoid private investigator equals, nothing to worry about! You should be happy!"

"I just—thinking back on it, the timing was impeccable—somebody called me right when the shots—whatever—went off."

"Then they were probably at the lake, too."

"But then they're following Fancy and me right? That's fucked up!"

"But they aren't shooting at you and Fancy! Good news!" Tammy's genuinely exasperated. Too exasperated to do me any more favors. But she might not be fed up with a certain terrier.

"No matter what, this guy called from this number, threatening Fancy. It's great that he didn't shoot at us, but still. I pick up Fancy today and now, now I don't think Fancy will be safe until we know . . ."

"Of course I'll trace the number. Shit, was that all you wanted? I assumed you had your own ju-jitsu for that. Write it down. I'll get back to you this afternoon. Wow, you're new at this crime stuff, huh?" Tammy's payment for this favor begins immediately, as I give her a look that rivals gluten-free vegan pizza for pathos. "I'll let you know this afternoon, Pran. Get your dog!"

———

Just when I though the Oakland Police Department had found every way to fail, a sliver of light: Tammy's parking validation actually works, and I sail from Broadway to the 980 with just enough time to rinse off my two-day yoga slime before I meet with its sponsor, Aria Butler.

I never had an aversion to oxymorons until I was exposed to essential oils. Even with the encouragement of hot water and soap, my skin is almost as embedded. Each layer reveals a new odor. Sweat, then an essential oil, then—more essential oil? Is this what verbena smells like?

I give myself just enough time to run into Trader Joe's for a shot of coffee to power me into Butch's Bucha Bar. Under threat of losing my vag badge, I have avoided Butch's. Kombucha might as well be sock-flavored Snapple as far as I'm concerned, but Aria likes what she likes. I sneak past several verbena-scented dervishes and ease through the door.

"Perfect! Prana, come here!" Aria gestures to me, resplendent in an orange caftan that somehow makes her look even taller, five people back from the front of a line that I now realize was the cause of the cluster around the entrance. I get snide side-eye from eight vested, sweatshirted, sensibly-coifed women behind Aria, arrayed two-by-two as if boarding an ark designed to repopulate an REI and a tea dance. "Do you know what you want? I always get the same thing."

The menu is separated into Butch's Bucha and Butch's Hoocha. I look at my watch and decide that I should probably order from the Bucha side, though the "+/- 24% ABV" makes the Hoocha seem mighty appealing. It's technically lunch time, after all. "Foodwise, what do you recommend?"

"Oh, I guess the Beetbeatdown, with a progurt booster? I don't usually eat until I'm done practicing for the day—maybe if my mula bandha was a little stronger—but don't let that stop you. People really like the wraps and the Mac'n'Cheer looks awesome. If only they were open after six." Aria sighs deeply.

"Hey Butch, wants some bucha?" Our handsome cashier, wearing a nametag that says "Butch Sara" makes this greeting sound as natural as tea rotting in a jar.

"Sure Butch, can I get a medium JazzyRazz for here and" Aria gestures at me.

"I'll get, um, a small MoscowMula?" Aria stares at me, obviously impressed at my adventurous ordering. "Also, um, is that kale-chips in the nachos?"

"Super-Slathered? You betcha, Butch."

"I'll get those, too." I wave my hand at Aria in the international gesture for "I'll pay for this" and pull out a ten and a twenty.

"Okay Butch, that'll be forty-one sixty-two." I hand over a credit card. "And this will help Butch find you when it's ready." I'm handed a picture of kd lang in a metal stand. By the time I sign my receipt, Aria's already found a spot for us at one of the two long communal tables.

"Thank you!" I pick up one of the cups of water Aria procured for us. "Is this silt?"

"Isn't it great? Earth-filtered." Aria's gulp leaves a faint mudstache on her upper lip. "So. How's my family?"

"Well." I hand her a spreadsheet. "The numbers add up, but they're only as reliable as the person entering them."

"All I care about," Aria slaps her right hand above her heart, the first time I've seen this gesture invested with any sincerity, "are my people. What do you know?"

"Your instincts are right on, but things are pretty, well, innocent. Michelle's the reason that the pouch seems to contract and expand. She's got, um, a sideline."

"Not bartending? I offered her hours, but she said she wasn't doing that anymore."

"No, way better. Have you ever been to 'Boom'?"

"Is that a dance club? I can't really go out after ten; I start fasting for morning practice at seven. But I love to dance. Do they have a tea dance?"

"It's a burlesque show. It's going on for a while, but they just moved across the bay, maybe," I calculate the last time I went with Iris, God, five months? "Boom"'s first show at the Stork? "Probably six months ago. Anyway, Michelle is the producer, Chica Boom. She's great, she dances, she's mean to the crowd. You'd love it. Anyway, she brings in all this cash in small bills and then changes it during savasana."

"But she's not stealing?"

"No—actually based on the data I got from your point-of-sale, I think she might be putting money in. Weird, right?"

"Her practice is so powerful. Should I talk to her?"

"I leave that to you."

"Her practice is REALLY powerful. Thank you, I am Jazzy." Aria points her chin alerting me to Butch Brie's stare.

"Yep, nachos." Butch Brie is unmoved. "I am . . . Super-Slathered." Butch Brie smiles and slides a small plate that looks like yard waste in front of me. It smells like leaves and salt. "Thanks."

"I'll be back with your MoscowMula!"

Aria takes a big swig of her kombucha. "I'm terrified of Michelle."

"Do you want to fire her for giving you money?"

"No. I think she's the best. Probably better than everyone else. But, I mean, I hired you, and now I know what's up, so I should do something, right?"

"That's not all." Apparently Butch Brie's allowed to give me my drink unacknowledged. It smells like old leaves and sugar. The woman sitting next to me can probably smell my drink, too. If it had a straw, she could probably lean in a grab a sip. I glance at my phone and see that Tammy has not forsaken me. "New post 27+ shares! Your caller: Raina Galvez. Kisses!"

I send a quick text to Aria suggesting that communal table might not be the best place to explain everything I've discovered about her employees, but Aria's still staring intently at me, too focused on working out Yoginitini's future to check her phone.

"What's not all? What else did you find?"

"Don't you want to check your phone?"

"What? No, I'm having lunch. Why?"

"Okay." The woman on my left's breath smells like old leaves and lemons. I glance at Aria's JazzyRazz, which is nearly finished. "We should go for a walk."

"But you have to eat. That looks so good. It's taking all my willpower not to dive into the chips, but y'know, cashews are legumes."

"Of course" I say, completely oblivious to the dangerous game each cashew plays, masquerading as a nut. I drain my MoscowMula. "Let's stroll! Do you like rat terriers?"

———

Aria is a human with feelings. Obviously she likes rat terriers. We head toward Iris's building to pick up Fancy. In addition to rat terriers, Aria also likes Tai, who apparently took Aria aside to spew compliments about me. "I think maybe she's got a crush? I came by on Tuesday after you'd left and she could not STOP talking about how open your hips are. She's like, 'Prana settled into pigeon like it was child's pose.'"

"How does she talk about most of her clients?" I suddenly reconsider the moment I caught her staring during savasana, the fight with her little suitor in the alley, her interest in knowing which studios I'd been to. Am I blushing?

"She doesn't. For a second I thought maybe you told her who you were and what you were doing there. I was so relieved, but then it turned out she just wanted to talk about your practice."

"Relieved?"

Aria stops and stares down, almost kicks some goose poop from the path and then stills her foot, toe digging into packed beige dirt. "I hate this. I hate keeping secrets. I mean, I guess everyone else is keeping secrets, too. I mean, is Tai . . . a problem?"

"She's teaching around a lot, but that's no secret. I haven't sniffed out anything yet, but I can look into her personal stuff. She probably has private clients that, um, make things easier."

"I kind of assumed she had some sort of situation. What about Faryn? I've been a little concerned. He's not, like, a rent boy or—"

"God no. He probably has a rent boy. Do you know where he lives?" Aria's too classy to pry, even as I expose the diverse economic realities allowing her employees to survive as yoga teachers in the bay area without stealing from her. She does not know where Faryn lives, but once I describe it, her shoulders slip even farther down her back, if possible, visible eased, her stroll becoming a saunter. If there's support Faryn needs that he's not getting from Yoginitini, it is manifestly not financial in nature.

"This is the end of it, right? I mean, I hired you, you figured out why the cash situation was weird, I've been a responsible business person . . . "

Do I tell Aria about the creepy stares, the phone call? Daryl Hall, never a team player, cuts off my train of thought, chiming from my pocket, "I see you! You see me!"

"Oh Prana, do you need to get that?" I shut him down without removing my phone from my vest.

"No, it's cool." I suddenly need this meeting to take place near a reliably unsoiled public bathroom. "Let's actually head the other way." I may need to shift from a saunter to a sprint. What is in a MoscowMula? Aria matches my pace without comment. "So, umm, are these the answers you hired me to get? Michelle's trafficking in small bills that she may not declare to the IRS?"

"Faryn's a trustafarian."

"Probably."

"And Tai—I mean, this is none of my business, is it? My husband's super-invested in Yoginitini being like, a serious capitalist *enterprise*. But it's not a start-up, it's not a tech incubator, I 've been thinking about it, and it's a home. For me, for everyone who wants the most inspiring, transformative teachers . . . and wine and artisanal cocktails." I nod. I feel like releasing enough breath to affirm her verbally might result in an unfortunate release between my sit bones. If I'm walking too fast for Aria, she hasn't mentioned it. "So maybe, yeah. Maybe I'm done?" She stops walking. I'm not sure if I can stand still. She faces me, a hand on each of my shoulders. "But I *love* your energy, Prana. Invoice me for the week, but then, just keep coming. You can come to my classes now!"

"I will. I will. I've gotta run. Is that okay?"

"Of course. Invoice me! And remember what you're worth when you do, Prana, this has been great!"

I start running.

———

If Trader Joe's on Lakeshore had predated Disneyland, Walt would never have been able to call his park the "Happiest Place on Earth" with a straight face. With my tiny paper cup of coffee from free sample corner (Joe's Café! Always Joe's treat!) and clear, empty bowels, I can settle into the elation of a job well done. I have a real, honest-to-God, satisfied customer that I didn't even go to college with. Aria sounded worried that my bill would be too small! I didn't have to wait for in line for the bathroom! I grab a bag of dark chocolate peanut butter cups, a trusted, stable energy source to replace whatever it was that just rejected me as a host, when I hear a familiar, "Yo Pran!"

Jen waves to me from the middle of the line. "Get up here!"

"Done for the day?"

"Nah, just for the moment. I've got a 'TJIP' session at four."

" 'TJI' "—

" 'Thank Joseph, It's Pilates.' It's funnier if you're obsessed with having a pelvic floor strong enough to shell a walnut. Anyway, it's pretty popular. But I'm done at seven. Wanna hang out? Jomer Jimpson and I were just going to watch some HGTV if you want to come over."

"Maybe. I'm picking up Fancy right now, but otherwise I didn't have any plans."

"You know who has a rat terrier who looks just like Fancy? That teacher from Yoginitini, Siam."

"You mean Tai?" We scooch forward, almost at the registers.

"That sounds right. Yeah, I just saw her and her pocket-sized boyfriend near the lake." Jen says and she sets out her bags, finally at the promised land, greeted by an adorable boy in a Hawaiian shirt.

"Huh." Could Tai have a rat terrier, too? We're always so quick to judge the people most like ourselves.

"I'll pay for these." Jen smiles at the cashier, and tosses me my cups. "Go to Fancy, Prana. You belong together." I blow Jen a kiss, pocket full of dark chocolate goodness, bound for Lake Merritt and a very special rat terrier, longing join me on a promenade.

———

I shove half the peanut butter cups in my face so fast that I give a quick shout out of gratitude to Joe the Trader, who, in his infinite wisdom, allows his cups to be unclothed by foil as God (or Joseph Pilates) intended. My vision becomes sharper, my steps firmer. By the time I enter Iris's building, I'm ready for another full turn around the lake with a double back for sniffing and groundtreats.

"Good afternoon." A stranger greets me. Something is wrong.

"Hey, I'm here to pick up Fancy. Iris's rat terrier?"

"Ms. Freidman's dog? There must be some confusion. Her co-parent already came by."

"What? I'm her—excuse me." Could Rafa be the little fellow Tai was fighting with in the alley? Are they walking Fancy right now? I barely glance at traffic before I bolt across the street to the lake. As I sprint south I think I can see two Tai and Rafa-shaped people and one Fancy, balking, but generally progressing north and west across the pedestrian bridge. I crouch low behind a shrub and try to hear Michelle's voice in my head, squeezing my legs into my chest. The rest of my cups fall from my vest pocket, but I let them be. I have all the peanut butter and chocolate I need to get my Fancy back.

When Fancy comes into sight I kick back and roll forward, a proud warrior that has just knocked Fancy's leash from Rafa's hand. "What the—Prana?" Tai looks confused, while Rafa scrambles behind me.

"You'll have to excuse me. Fancy and I have places to be."

"Oh yeah?" Rafa waves a dark chocolate peanut butter cup.

"You don't eat those Fancy! Fancy!" she lunges toward Rafa's sinister offering. "Fancy, OOPS." She turns to me and I grab her leash, thankful there are any commands that could compel a heart so free. "Oh Fancy! The fuck were you thinking, Rafa?"

"Don't look at me. It was Tai's idea."

Tai holds her head in her hands, seated on the grass. "Fuck you, Prana. Just walk in, with your open hips, flashing your perfect dog and your perfect name. So we wanted to walk your dog, so what!"

Rafa tosses the cups into the lake. "She's lying. Don't look at me! I'm not protecting you anymore! She's been off the rails for months, then she saw you at the studio, at the lake."

"What?" I can't believe Tai ever noticed us checking out her class. Tai looks at me, pale, not flushed, as if she no longer has the energy for shame.

"Oh what, you think *everybody* can get their hips to the floor in pigeon? Everyone just pops into camel on the first try? Fuck you, Prana. Why were you even watching me? Like I could have anything to give—" Rafa puts one arm around Tai, offering the peanut butter cup to her with the other. "You know peanuts are legumes, Rafa!" As she finishes she snatches the cup from his hands with her mouth and collapse into him, chewing slowly.

Rafa strokes Tai hair for a moment. Directing himself at Fancy, who returns his gaze between sniffing at the dirt for any struggle-produced chocolate particulates, Rafa sighs. "Just got fixated, I guess. I mean, I'd told her about Fancy, and then, when we figured out who you were." Rafa shakes a weary horizontal mustache.

"But it's just yoga, man. Fancy is my partner. Why, why would you ever?"

"Tai's been off for a while, and there was no way—she can't be well here, I mean she can barely eat. When it was obvious that you were messing with her, I just thought, fuck it. We're leaving. Back to Washington. And we're taking your little dog, too. I know it sounds crazy."

"Messing with her? What?"

Tai looks up. "Come on. Private lessons. Just rubbing my nose in it! Some one like that, you don't deserve . . . "

I look at Fancy. Tai shakes, brushing away tears. I will never know how miserable her life was, I think, trying to make a living teaching yoga in the East Bay. Fancy snuffles at my leg. I will never know what it's like to live without the love of a rat terrier, but I get a strange sensation that it's like that pose where you sit on your foot, but instead of jamming your heel into your ass, you smash it in your heart. "Rafa. Did you let Fancy eat anything weird from the ground?"

"No. NO. And I wouldn't have let her eat the cup either . . . I just . . . Tai needs to get over herself, you know. I thought this would be it."

"And you're leaving."

"I'm about to hand over my savings for a Civic, then we're out of here tomorrow. Back to Renton. Please, Prana. Does this have to be a thing?"

I look at Fancy. I look at the lake. If anyone can afford to be generous, it's Prana Weinberg, MA, PHR, PI.

Saturday

Like they were ever going to start over in a Civic. Tai and Rafa's baggage requires a Honda Accord. We conduct our business on the porch, in the olfactory range of so many sweet and savory barbecues that Fancy might be too paralyzed by choice to run off in one direction or the other, so she tugs insistently at my leggings to let me know that she requires my input. As I sign over Zsa Zsa's title, I note Rafa's signature. R, squiggle, Galvez with the tail of the "z" stretching down, like Fancy's tail on a cold, wet constitutional before I found her booties. Identical, I imagine, to his signature when the "R" stood for "Raina." Rafa comes alone. He pauses after handing over the four-thousand dollar cashier's check and looks longingly at Fancy.

"You know, she's so beautiful. But crazy. Crazy!"

"Fancy just knows what she likes. It doesn't have to be good for her."

Rafa laughs. "No, Tai. She thinks everything's a dance company—ten principals, twelve soloists, twenty in the corps. At Yoginitini, she's a principal. Then you come in. Kind of old, lumpy, know nothing" I nod, so that Rafa knows I can hear him. Still, for four grand I've heard worse. "but so fucking good at yoga. So spirited. You share custody of one of Iris Isersmilink's dogs!" Rafa smooths his mustache. "It's like, you showed her that there's no meritocracy, you can work as hard as you want, but then someone will just show up with better, um, *prana.*" I pick up Fancy and nod. Rafa gives her a final scratch behind her left ear.

"Good luck. Take care of her." Rafa walks away before I can decide if I want to return the sentiment. I nuzzle Fancy, put her down, and open the front door.

"Who wants to write an invoice? Who wants to write an invoice?" She lets me trudge to my office on my own. As I calculate my mileage for the past six days, I find a treat in the pocket of the vest hanging off the back of my chair.

"Oops!"

Fancy's collar rattles as she ascends the stairs. "Excellent tracking and capture, partner."

Fancy looks up at me, treat already apprehended and consumed. "I'll see that our rate reflects your efforts."

Fancy glares. Promises sound good, but they don't smell like organ meat. I give her another treat, and a scratch, whether she deserves it or not. It's what you do for your partner when you need her on the next case.

The End

About the Author

Margaret France teaches yoga and literature in Rock Island, Illinois. Her spirit animal is Dolly Parton.

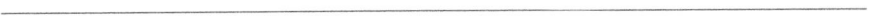

www.ingramcontent.com/pod-product-compliance
Lightning Source LLC
Chambersburg PA
CBHW032122280326
41933CB00009B/947